# Patient Safety
## Emerging Applications of Safety Science

**Claire Cox**
**Helen Hughes**
**Jordan Nicholls**

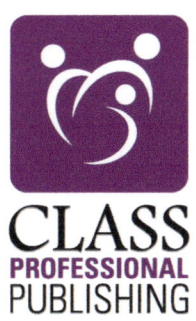

Class Professional Publishing have made every effort to ensure that the information, tables, drawings and diagrams contained in this book are accurate at the time of publication. The book cannot always contain all the information necessary for determining appropriate care and cannot address all individual situations; therefore, individuals using the book must ensure they have the appropriate knowledge and skills to enable suitable interpretation. Class Professional Publishing does not guarantee, and accepts no legal liability of whatever nature arising from or connected to, the accuracy, reliability, currency or completeness of the content of *Patient Safety: Emerging Applications of Safety Science*. Users must always be aware that such innovations or alterations after the date of publication may not be incorporated in the content. Please note, however, that Class Professional Publishing assumes no responsibility whatsoever for the content of external resources in the text or accompanying online materials.

Text © Claire Cox, Helen Hughes and Jordan Nicholls 2024

All rights reserved. Without limiting the rights under copyright reserved above, no part of this publication may be reproduced, stored in or introduced into a retrieval system, or transmitted, in any form or by any means (electronic, mechanical, photocopying, recording or otherwise) without the prior written permission of the publisher of this book.

The information presented in this book is accurate and current to the best of the authors' knowledge. The authors and publisher, however, make no guarantee as to, and assume no responsibility for, the correctness, sufficiency or completeness of such information or recommendation.

The authors and publisher welcome feedback from the users of this book. Please contact the publisher:

Class Professional Publishing,
The Exchange, Express Park, Bristol Road, Bridgwater TA6 4RR

Telephone: 01278 472 800
Email: info@class.co.uk
Website: www.classprofessional.co.uk

Class Professional Publishing is an imprint of Class Publishing Ltd
A CIP catalogue record for this book is available from the British Library

Paperback ISBN: 9781801610834
ePub ISBN: 9781801610841
ePDF ISBN: 9781801610858

Cover design by Nicky Borowiec
Designed and typeset by PHi Business Solutions
Printed in the UK by Hobbs

This book is printed on paper from responsible sources. Refer to local recycling guidance on disposal of this book.

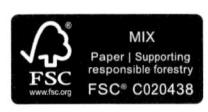
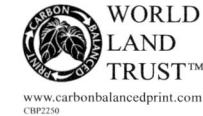

# Contents

Contributors Biographies — ix
Foreword — xix
*Ted Baker*

List of Abbreviations — xxi

## 1  Introduction — 1
*Claire Cox, Jordan Nicholls and Helen Hughes*

Patient Safety in the NHS — 1
Practical Tools for Patient Safety — 2
Engagement with Patients and Families — 3
Proactive Safety within Healthcare — 3
References — 4

## 2  The Theory of Change Management and its Application in Quality and Safety — 5
*Julie Storr*

Summary — 5
Background — 5
The Theory Behind Change Management — 6
    Change Management Outside of Healthcare — 6
    Change Management within the Healthcare System — 7
Improving the Safety of Care Delivery — A Universal Challenge — 9
Examples of Change Management and Patient Safety in a Complex System — 11
    The Importance of Leadership — 11
    Change, Implementation and Improvement — 11
    Application of Change Management Principles to Patient Safety — 12
    A Practical Framework for Change Management — the NHS Change Model — 14
Conclusion — 14
References — 15

## 3 The Systems Engineering Initiative for Patient Safety (SEIPS): A Human Factors Approach to Work System Analysis   19
*Paul Bowie and Helen Vosper*

| | |
|---|---|
| Summary | 19 |
| Background | 19 |
| The SEIPS Framework Explained | 20 |
| Examples of the Multi-functionality of SEIPS | 23 |
| SEIPS and Basic Systems Thinking Principles | 24 |
|     Comparison Between SEIPS and the Fishbone Diagram | 25 |
| Application of SEIPS: The NHS Health Check | 26 |
| Final Thoughts | 27 |
| **Case Study 1** Vicky Baker | 28 |
| **Case Study 2** Victoria Wills | 31 |
| **Case Study 3** Anonymous NHS Secondary Care Provider | 36 |
| Reflections from the Frontline | 38 |
| References | 39 |

## 4 Patient and Family Engagement Following Patient Safety Incidents   41
*Lauren Ramsey, Louise Pye and Jane O'Hara*

| | |
|---|---|
| Summary | 41 |
| Background | 41 |
|     Why is Patient and Family Engagement Following Patient Safety Incidents Important? | 41 |
|     Meeting the Needs of Patients and Families Following Patient Safety Incidents — A Moral Duty? | 43 |
|     The Importance of the Patient and Family Perspective to Support Organisational Learning | 44 |
|     What is Compounded Harm? | 44 |
| What do We Already Know About Patient and Family Engagement Following Patient Safety Incidents? | 45 |
|     A Patient and Family Perspective | 46 |
|     A Clinician's Perspective | 46 |
|     An Engagement Lead's Perspective | 47 |
|     The Impact of Litigation | 50 |
|     The Impact of the Healthcare Setting | 50 |
|     Learn Together | 50 |
|     System-Level Challenges | 52 |
| What Could Patient and Family Engagement Following Patient Safety Incidents Look Like in the Future? | 53 |
|     What Can We Learn From Other Sectors? | 53 |
|     An International Perspective | 54 |
|     Innovations in Engagement | 55 |
|     Patient and Family Advocacy | 56 |
| Final Thoughts | 58 |
| **Case Study 1** Anonymous Patient Safety Manager from an Acute Trust | 58 |
| Reflections from the Frontline | 61 |
| References | 61 |

## 5 Safety-II — 65
*Mark Sujan*

| | |
|---|---|
| Summary | 65 |
| Background | 65 |
|    There is No Safety-I | 65 |
|    Why Do We Need Safety-II? | 66 |
|    What is Safety-II? | 67 |
| Applying Safety-II | 68 |
|    Understanding 'Work As Done' | 68 |
|    Learning from Everyday Work | 68 |
|    Challenges in the Application of Safety-II Thinking | 70 |
| Example of the Application of Safety-II in the Management of Deterioration | 70 |
| Final Thoughts | 72 |
| Acknowledgements | 72 |
| **Case Study 1** Anonymous Patient Safety Manager from an Acute Trust | 73 |
| Reflections from the Frontline | 77 |
| References | 77 |

## 6 After Action Review — 79
*Judy Walker*

| | |
|---|---|
| Summary | 79 |
| Background | 79 |
| The Theory Behind the Practice of AAR | 80 |
| The Five Components of the AAR | 82 |
|    The Four Questions | 82 |
|    Scoping the Specific Purpose of the AAR | 83 |
|    The AAR Conductor | 84 |
|    AAR Ground Rules | 85 |
|    Participants | 85 |
|    Patients and Family Members as Participants in AARs | 86 |
|    AAR Research | 86 |
| Implementation | 87 |
|    Quality Issues | 87 |
|    Legal Issues | 87 |
| Final Thoughts | 87 |
| **Case Study 1** Katy Fisher | 88 |
| **Case Study 2** Lisa Moss | 90 |
| Reflections from the Frontline | 92 |
| References | 93 |

## 7 Walk-Through-Talk-Through Analysis to Support Healthcare Safety and Improvement Activity — 95
*Richard Brownhill and Paul Bowie*

| | |
|---|---|
| Summary | 95 |
| Background | 95 |
| What is WT3? | 96 |
|    Anticipated Benefits of WT3 | 96 |
|    Performance Influencing Factors (PIFs) | 97 |
|    Exploring Human Work | 99 |

| | |
|---|---|
| How to Apply WT3 | 99 |
| Who Can Use WT3? | 100 |
| Key Questions and Prompts | 101 |
| Advantages and Disadvantages of WT3 | 102 |
| Other Considerations | 102 |
| Final Thoughts | 102 |
| Acknowledgements | 103 |
| **Case Study 1** Chris Elston and Kayleigh Edwards | 103 |
| Reflections from the Frontline | 108 |
| References | 108 |
| Reading | 108 |
| Appendix 1 | 110 |

## 8 AcciMaps — 113
*Jayne Wheway and Patrick Waterson*

| | |
|---|---|
| Summary | 113 |
| Background | 113 |
| Steps to Construct an AcciMap | 114 |
| ActorMaps | 124 |
| Final Thoughts | 125 |
| Acknowledgements | 125 |
| **Case Study 1** Wendy Halliburton | 125 |
| **Case Study 2** Chris Elston | 131 |
| Reflections from the Frontline | 135 |
| References | 136 |

## 9 Transformative Simulation: To Patient Safety and Beyond — 139
*Philip Gurnett, Sharon Weldon, Ken Spearpoint and Andy Buttery*

| | |
|---|---|
| Summary | 139 |
| Background | 139 |
| Simulation in Other Industries | 141 |
| Human Factors and Ergonomics (HFE) and Its Link to Transformative Simulation | 141 |
| The Transformative Simulation Taxonomy | 142 |
| Application | 143 |
| Conclusions | 146 |
| **Case Study 1** Emma Broughton | 146 |
| Reflections from the Frontline | 151 |
| References | 151 |

## 10 Thematic Reviews in Patient Safety — 155
*Samantha Machen*

| | |
|---|---|
| Summary | 155 |
| Background | 155 |
| The Argument for Thematic Reviews | 156 |
| When to Do a Thematic Review? | 158 |
| How to Do a Thematic Review of Patient Safety Incidents | 158 |

    Who Should be Conducting Thematic Reviews? 158
    What Data Can be Used Within a Thematic Review of Patient Safety Incidents? 159
    What are the Minimum Data Standards for Inclusion in a Thematic Review? 159
    How Can Data be Analysed? 160
    How Many Incidents or Cases Do I Need to Include in the Thematic Review? 160
    How Long Does a Thematic Review Take? 160
Example of How a Thematic Review Can be Used 161
Final Thoughts 162
**Case Study 1** Andy Wilmer 162
Reflections from the Frontline 166
References 166

# 11 Conclusion 169
*Claire Cox, Jordan Nicholls and Helen Hughes*

References 171

# Contributors Biographies

**Andy Buttery**, after 20 years' clinical work as an Operating Department Practitioner (ODP), developed an increased interest in education and improvement which led to a full-time educator role as Simulation Specialist in 2004. He was a Human Factors Editor for the European Simulation Conference (SESAM) in 2014 and 2015 and is the European subject expert for the initial working group on the International Certification as Healthcare Simulation Educator (CHSE) award. He co-designed and delivered a workshop on Human Factors Education for the UK Clinical Human Factors Group in 2012. He has lapsed qualifications as a RC(UK) ALS Instructor and GIC Faculty; ACLS Provider; TeamSTEPPS Master Trainer; Simulated Patient Framework SP and SP Trainer; CHSE; and is a co-author of a few papers.

Now Regional Simulation and Human Factors Project Lead for Health Education England South East (HEE KSS), Andy's role is largely managerial and developmental, although he still manages to sneak out and teach on occasion. He is confident that simulation-based education will continue to evolve and provide elegant, effective solutions to challenges in health and care.

**Andy Wilmer** works at King's College Hospital NHS Foundation Trust as the Associate Director of Patient Safety. He has worked at King's since 2012 in several patient safety, patient experience and quality governance roles. He has a particular interest in systems thinking in patient safety and has led the organisation's implementation of the NHS Patient Safety Incident Response Framework.

**Callum Brown** is a pharmacist by background who now works full-time in Patient Safety and Experience. Callum's main areas of expertise are the disciplines of Patient Safety and Quality Improvement, and his main area of interest is how these two disciplines can be linked to improve the safety and experience of not only patients but healthcare staff also. Callum has worked in these disciplines in various NHS Trusts and other organisations and has a wealth of knowledge spanning the entire healthcare system. Callum holds a PgCert in Patient Safety and Quality Improvement, MSc in Health and Care System Leadership and is a Chartered Manager.

**Charlotte Overton** is Research Fellow with the Yorkshire and Humber Patient Safety Research Collaboration. Her research interests include the use of social science theories and qualitative methods in implementation science and patient safety research and the translation of policy into practice. She is also a practising acute care nurse and has previously worked as researcher-in-residence.

**Chris Elston** spent 24 years in the Royal Navy, starting as a medical assistant in shore establishments and joining the submarine service upon completion of his initial training. This increased his scope of practice to include atmosphere control and radiation protection, including radiochemistry and nuclear monitoring. Finding a passion for teaching his career took him back to the medical schools where he taught on the Royal Navy specific components of medical assistant training at the Defence Medical Services Training Centre. In 2001, he commenced his nursing training at the University of Central England in Birmingham, as part of the first military course to undertake training at this university, specialising in Emergency Care at MDHU Portsmouth (at the Queen Alexandra Hospital) and being deployed with the Royal Marines to operations in Afghanistan. Returning to the education arena, he was drafted back to the Defence Medical Services Training Group, instructing on the common core programme of the defence medics course, with a remit for developing and supporting trainees that required additional support to complete the course. Since leaving the Royal Navy, Chris has been employed as a charge nurse in ED and the IV devices nurse with a large safety brief. Developing his interest in human factors he studied Applied Ergonomics and Human Factors, before joining the University Hospital Southampton NHS Foundation Trust as the Patient Safety Education Lead.

**Claire Cox** is an experienced nurse of over 25 years. She has worked in numerous specialities in the NHS and in different places around the world, from being a repatriation nurse to volunteering in refugee camps and striking up collaborations with nurses in America. Claire's most recent clinical role was as a Critical Care Outreach Sister 2011–2020, where her desire for patient safety was ignited. After winning the Kent Surrey and Sussex Patient Safety Prize in 2016 for her work in cardiac arrest and medical emergency teams, Claire went on to complete the Darzi fellowship (clinical leadership) in April 2019. Following this fellowship, Claire started working with the charity, Patient Safety Learning. This gave Claire insight and contacts with leaders from inside and outside of the NHS. In September 2020, Claire began an exciting new career in patient safety at Guy's and St Thomas' Hospital NHS Foundation Trust. This gave Claire a great foundation of how patient safety is managed within the largest NHS trust in the UK. Claire currently works at King's College Hospital NHS Foundation Trust where she is currently a Clinical Patient Safety Lead. This is an exciting role as she is helping to shape and embed the new Patient Safety Incident Response Framework within the Trust. Claire co-founded and chairs the Patient Safety Management Network in June 2021. This network has grown to nearly 1600 members nationwide and meets weekly to discuss the evolving management of patient safety. The purpose of this network is to collaborate, learn together, share and provide peer support.

**Deb Hazeldine** was compelled to take on a very public, central role in campaign efforts for a Public Inquiry into the Mid Staffordshire disaster after witnessing the heart-breaking, unnecessary suffering and death of her mother at Mid Staffordshire Hospital in 2006. She gave evidence to the Health Care Commission, on oath to the Robert Francis Mid Staffs Public Inquiry, and in December 2018 was awarded an MBE for her services to patient safety in Staffordshire. Having witnessed the investigation process, she is very passionate about patients and families having a voice and being heard in all aspects of NHS care and investigations.

**Emma Broughton** is a paediatric nurse and clinical educator, currently working as the Head of Education for Simulation at Great Ormond Street Hospital. She completed her MSc in Health and Medical Simulation at the University of Hertfordshire, graduating in 2022. Emma is passionate about using simulation to create learning experiences that are innovative, engaging and meaningful; from rehearsing events alongside teams in their clinical environment, to using simulation to inform and influence practice. Emma has a particular interest in the application of simulation to improve clinical practice and foster a safer environment for patients and staff.

**Helen Hughes** is Chief Executive of Patient Safety Learning. Helen's passion for improved patient safety is informed by personal family insight into the impact of unsafe care and the ineffectiveness of organisational responses to learn from error. Helen is an experienced leader in organisational effectiveness and transformational change. She has held leadership roles in healthcare in the UK and the WHO, the National Patient Safety Agency, Equality and Human Rights Commission, Parliamentary Health Services Ombudsman and the Charity Commission. Helen's previous leadership roles in patient safety include, as Director of Operations of the National Patient Safety Agency, designing the first patient safety infrastructure and policy framework for the NHS in England, and Director of the National Reporting and Learning System. At the WHO, she held a range of roles, including partnership and patient safety programme management and executive lead of the global 'Patients For Patient Safety' programme.

**Helen Vosper** is a chartered Human Factors specialist and graduate of the Loughborough Human Factors Masters Programme. Helen is an experienced educator with extensive experience of teaching Human Factors to healthcare students and professionals. She is currently the lead for Patient Safety in the Institute of Education in Healthcare and Medical Sciences at the University of Aberdeen. Helen also has a part-time role as a Senior Investigation Science Educator at the Health Services Safety Investigations Body (HSSIB) and is a scientific adviser in Human Factors and Patient Safety to NHS Education for Scotland.

**Jacqui Evans** has worked at the York and Scarborough Teaching Hospitals NHS Foundation Trust since 2021. She is a Registered Nurse (Oxford) and holds a BSc (Hons) in Management and Systems and a MPhil in systems methodology applied to risk management (both City University). She previously worked at a senior level in acute healthcare in Hertfordshire for almost 20 years having various roles with managerial responsibility for patient safety, quality improvement and clinical governance. She developed a strong appreciation for family engagement and involvement while supporting families through investigations, complaints, claims and inquests. In 2021 the hills and seaside beckoned, and Jacqui relocated to North Yorkshire. Her current role is split between undertaking Patient Safety Incident Investigations and supporting the patient safety team with emerging projects.

**Jane O'Hara** is Director of Research at The Healthcare Improvement Studies (THIS) Institute, at the University of Cambridge. She leads the Safer Systems, Cultures and Practices theme within the NIHR Yorkshire & Humber Patient Safety Research Collaboration (running 2023–2028) and leads a large NIHR-funded programme evaluating the Patient Safety Incident Response Framework (May 2022–July 2025). Jane also holds Visiting Professor positions at the University of Leeds, and the SHARE Centre for Resilience in Healthcare at the University of Stavanger, Norway. She has nearly fifteen years' experience leading patient safety research, and a further eight years of applied psychological research prior to that. Jane has received funding from THIS Institute, the Trondheim Foundation and Research Council of Norway, and the NIHR Programme Grants for Applied Health Research, and the NIHR Policy Research Unit programme. Jane has a broad range of research interests including engaging patients and families in care quality and safety; measurement and monitoring of patient safety; safety theory and resilient healthcare approaches; co-production; and quality and safety intervention development and testing.

**Jayne Wheway** is Patient Safety Clinical Lead for Children's, Young People and Human Factors in the National Patient Safety Team at NHS England. Jayne has been a Registered Nurse (Mental Health) for more than 30 years. She has a BSc (Hons) in Advanced Professional Practice from the University of Nottingham, an MSc in Health Services Management from King's College London, and an MSc in Ergonomics and Human Factors for Patient Safety from Loughborough University. She is also a Chartered Ergonomist/Human Factors Specialist. Jayne is a faculty member of the Chartered Institute of Ergonomics and Human Factors (CIEHF) accredited Healthcare Pathway for Human Factors for Patient Safety, and the Patient Safety Syllabus training for the NHS, both led by Loughborough University. She is proud to have been part of national projects such as the oversight and delivery boards for the NHS England, Royal

College of Paediatrics and Child Health, and Royal College of Nursing work on the National Paediatric Early Warning System, the NHS England Cross-system Sepsis Programme Board, and several National Patient Safety Alerts. Jayne's practice and research interests are in systems models for patient safety, including for spotting and acting on deterioration, multiple incident investigation and for national learning.

**Jordan Nicholls** has worked in patient safety across a number of sectors, including paediatric care, mental health and the ambulance service. With a degree in Drama, Applied Theatre and Education from the Royal Central School of Speech and Drama, Jordan has focussed on how to identify key learning for different healthcare audiences, and aiming to develop new and innovative ways of reducing the systemic risks of incidents reoccurring. Before working in patient safety, Jordan started his career in the busy press offices of both the ambulance and police services. He uses this communications background to help with engaging staff and patients in key safety topics. During the Covid-19 pandemic, Jordan created 'EEAST General Broadcast', a podcast that promoted safety in the prehospital sector by speaking to national and international experts, when engaging with staff face to face was difficult. Jordan is a trained QSIR practitioner and completed a QI coaching course to support teams in embedding safety practices. He is also a mental health first aider, with a focus on reducing the impact on second and third victims of incidents. He has a particular interest in Human Factors and Ergonomics, which helps to steer how best to embed safe practices into patient care. Jordan is an advocate of the Patient Safety Managers Network, noting that it is a key part of his work routine to engage with other safety professionals to work together.

**Judy Walker** is an After Action Review Conductor and Trainer working for a private company with clients across the world in healthcare, higher education, the World Health Organization, legal and corporate business settings. She was one of the first users of After Action Review in the NHS when employed by University College London Hospitals NHS Foundation Trust (UCLH) in 2008 where she conducted many AARs and trained hundreds of AAR Conductors. She has written and published regularly on the topic. Between 2015 and 2019, Judy worked as an Organisational Development Consultant as part of the Healthcare Consultancy team at NHS North East London Commissioning Support Unit. Her diverse portfolio of work there included designing a bespoke education programme for clinicians to improve end of life care, increasing staff engagement in large teams and coaching teams through change processes. Judy has a BA (Hons) in Education and Social Biology and qualifications as an ILM level 5 Coach, Hospital Play Specialist, NHS Train the Trainer, MBTI and Belbin Assessor. Her career began as a pioneer Hospital Play Specialist (HPS) in 1986 at St Stephen's Hospital, the Middlesex Hospital (1988) and later UCLH, transforming the quality and safety of paediatric services. She grew the play service from one individual employed as an HPS (herself) to 18 staff, ensuring all patients from birth to 18 years received developmentally appropriate support in the healthcare setting. She championed children's right to play in hospital nationally in her role as Chairman of the National Association of Hospital Play Staff and wrote the book "Play for Health" in 2006.

**Julie Storr** is a director and co-founder at KS Healthcare Consulting and has an international portfolio of work, including working currently as a senior technical expert with the World Health Organization. Her areas of focus include leading on the development, implementation and evaluation of guidelines and implementation-related resources in the field of patient safety, quality, antimicrobial resistance, Water, Sanitation and Hygiene (WASH), and infection prevention and control. She was previously President of the Infection Prevention Society of the UK and Ireland, Assistant Director at the English National Patient Safety Agency, and Director of the award winning national 'cleanyourhands' campaign. Change management theory and its practical application in the field is central to her day-to-day work. Julie is an honorary advisor at Tropical Health Education Trust and a steering group member of Health Information for

All. She is also a trained clinical hypnotherapist. Julie is the author of two books, most recently *Infection prevention and control: a social science perspective*, and has published widely in the academic literature.

**Katy Fisher** is currently Senior Nurse (Quality and Improvement) at NHS Professionals. After starting her career as an Adult Registered Nurse practicing in acute stroke, acute neurology, complex discharge planning and general medical nursing, she progressed to lead clinical governance, quality and risk management frameworks in acute hospitals in the Greater Manchester region. Her main interests are psychological safety as a system and creating learning and improvement processes within the healthcare setting. She has led acute patient safety collaboratives, conducted complex multi-disciplinary After Action Reviews and has led numerous high level patient safety investigations focussing on both Safety I and Safety II in formal clinical governance structures. She is passionate about making patient safety theory and methodology meaningful in a frontline healthcare setting.

**Kayleigh Edwards** is in her final year of her BSc Adult Nursing Degree, studying at Solent University in Southampton. Once qualified she hopes to work in palliative and end of life care. She is currently working for the Community Team at Mountbatten Hospice in Southampton alongside her studying.

**Ken Spearpoint** is an Associate Professor in Learning and Teaching; principal lecturer in medical simulation at the University of Hertfordshire and is the programme director of the MSc in Health and Medical Simulation. The application of human factors/ergonomics science to education and patient safety is integral to the programme. He has a particular interest in the integration of Safety II science into the design and delivery of clinical simulation and debriefing. Prior to taking up his position in academia in 2016, Ken worked in healthcare for more than 33 years. Ken is an intensive care trained nurse who worked in critical care in the NHS for 29 years, from 2004 he was a Nurse Consultant in Resuscitation at Imperial College Healthcare NHS Trust. Ken has a BSc (Hons) in Life Sciences, an MSc in Advanced Practice in Critical Care and an MPhil in Health Research. Ken has an established research and publication portfolio and has been involved in regional, national and international research initiatives in the field of resuscitation. He is a member of the Resuscitation Council UK research and development committee and an honorary life member of the Resuscitation Council UK.

**Lauren Ramsey** is a Senior Research Fellow based at the Yorkshire and Humber Patient Safety Research Collaboration (YH PSRC), England. Lauren has a broad range of research interests that centre on improving the quality and safety of care in the NHS. These interests include safety culture, patient involvement in patient safety, digital approaches to patient safety and safety inequities. More specifically, Lauren is a keen qualitative methodologist, with a particular interest in how such approaches can help to answer key research questions in these areas. Lauren has worked with the Yorkshire Quality and Safety Research (YQSR) group since 2013 and completed a PhD in 2020 with the University of Leeds and the Yorkshire and Humber Patient Safety Translational Research Centre (YH PSTRC) where she used an ethnographic approach to explore how healthcare staff respond to and use online patient feedback to improve the quality and safety of care. Since completing her PhD, Lauren has worked across various research projects which centre on the involvement of patients in patient safety, including the Learn Together programme, aiming to involve patients and families following patient safety incidents in healthcare more meaningfully. Most recently, Lauren works as a Senior Research Fellow within the theme of research titled, '*Safer Systems, Culture and Practices*' at the YH PSTRC.

**Lisa Moss** is a nurse with over 30 years' experience. She began her nurse training at King's College University in 1990 qualifying in 1993 and was in the second group of the newly formed

Project 2000 diploma. She began her nursing career at the then Bromley NHS Trust and worked initially on the medical wards and then went to the Intensive Care Unit at Bromley Hospital where she stayed for five years. In 2001 she joined Southwark primary care trust as a Nurse Advisor for NHS Direct. Having always had an interest in midwifery she began her midwifery training in 2003, qualifying in 2005 with a BSc. She specialised in high-risk midwifery and spent the last five years in the very privileged role of Specialist Bereavement midwife and set up the first Bereavement suite at the Princess Royal University Hospital, Farnborough. She went on to become a Supervisor of Midwives, and she was very proud to achieve the trust's 'Midwife of the year' award in 2014. Working in this role sparked her interest in patient safety and she joined the Patient Safety Team at Denmark Hill as a Patient Safety Lead in 2017. This is currently a very exciting time in Patient Safety with the roll out of the Patient Safety Incident Response Framework (PSIRF) and she is looking forward to helping embed these exciting changes in how patient safety incidents are responded to.

**Louise Pye** is the Head of Family Engagement for the Maternity and Newborn Safety Investigations (MNSI) programme. The programme was established in 2018 as part of the Healthcare Safety Investigation Branch (HSIB) and is now hosted by the Care Quality Commission (CQC). Describing the model of family engagement that was developed for HSIB, Lou was co-author of *Giving families a voice: HSIB's approach to patient and family engagement during investigations* and also a participating author in the NHSE guidance *Engaging and Involving patients, families and staff following patient safety incident*. Before she joined MNSI and HSIB, Lou served as an officer in the police force for 30 years, where she specialised in the field of family liaison. This involved working with families during serious and complex investigations.

**Mark Sujan** is a Chartered Ergonomist and Human Factors specialist (C.ErgHF). He has worked in patient safety and other safety-critical industries for over 25 years. Mark is Professor of Safety Science at the University of York, with a particular focus on safety assurance of systems involving artificial intelligence (AI) technologies.

In his role as Senior Investigation Science Educator at the Health Services Safety Investigations Body (HSSIB), Mark supports the delivery of core courses, including Patient Safety Incident Response Oversight and Demystifying Thematic Analysis. He also represents HSSIB in discussions and collaborations with other stakeholders regarding AI and Digital Health. Mark is a Trustee of the Chartered Institute of Ergonomics and Human Factors (CIEHF), which is the professional membership body for Human Factors and Ergonomics in the UK. He chairs the CIEHF special interest group on AI and Digital Health.

**Patrick Waterson** is Professor of Human Factors and Complex Systems at Loughborough University. During his career he has worked as a Research Fellow and MRC Scientist at Sheffield University (1992–2002) and Head of Department at the Fraunhofer Institute for Experimental Software Engineering in Germany (2002–2006). He joined Loughborough University in 2007. In 2014 he was awarded the William Floyd Medal from the UK Institute of Ergonomics and Human Factors for outstanding contribution to the field of Human Factors. In 2021 he was awarded the International Ergonomics Association (IEA)/Elsevier John Wilson Award 2021. The Award recognises major contributions in the field of applied ergonomics to the actual design of work, systems, technologies and environment, which lead to improvements in system performance and well-being.

**Paul Bowie** is currently Programme Director (Safety and Improvement) with NHS Education for Scotland based in Glasgow, Scotland, and he is also Professor of Human Factors for Health & Social Care at Staffordshire University. Paul is a chartered ergonomist and Human Factors expert, safety scientist and medical educator with over 30 years of experience leading and collaborating in research, innovation and educational development to improve the quality and safety of healthcare in the UK and globally. Paul is Honorary Professor and a PhD supervisor and examiner in the School of Health and Wellbeing at the University of Glasgow, and Adjunct Professor at Queen's University in Ontario, Canada. He is an Honorary Fellow of the Royal College of Physicians of Edinburgh and the Royal College of General Practitioners, and a Registered Member of the UK Chartered Institute of Ergonomics and Human Factors, where he is also the Healthcare Sector Group Lead on Patient Safety.

**Phil Gurnett** is a Clinical Simulation Fellow at the University of Greenwich. He has worked in healthcare simulation for nearly 10 years and has used simulation in both educational and non-educational approaches across a variety of healthcare settings. He qualified as a nurse in 2003 and has worked in cardiac and emergency care for the majority of that time. In 2017, he moved into simulation full time, running a hospital-based interprofessional simulation service as well as undertaking a PG cert in Ergonomics due to his passion for Human Factors/ergonomics. At this time, he also saw the value of simulation to identify latent threats to practice, delivering in situ simulation as a way to understand near miss events and to take training and development to clinical areas. During the COVID pandemic, in addition to the upskill training that was delivered by the team, they designed and delivered a simulation to understand how a vaccine service provision might look, the requirements for space and the system's requirements to deliver a successful service to the local healthcare economy. He moved to the University of Greenwich in 2021 where he took up the role of Clinical Simulation Fellow, supporting educational simulation and continuing to contribute to the development of transformative simulation. He continues to practice as a Resuscitation Officer and volunteers as a Community First Responder with his local ambulance service.

**Richard Brownhill** is a Head of Improvement for the Emergency Care Improvement Support Team at NHS England. Qualifying as a registered nurse in 1993, his experience has been mainly in emergency and acute care, working in senior nursing and operational roles. He has an MSc in advanced clinical practice and broadened his portfolio to work in general practice as a prescribing advanced practitioner, an urgent care commissioner and lecturer on the advanced practice programme. He has served on the NICE accreditation committee, the Royal College of Nursing emergency care association board, and the Royal College of Psychiatrists' PLAN committee, recognising the importance of needing shared principles across a complex system. As part of the chief nursing officer's safe staffing faculty, he has co-designed the emergency department safer nursing care tool (ED SNCT) and is currently studying for an MSc in human factors in patient safety and is a Clinical Human Factors Group Ambassador.

**Samantha Machen** is currently the Associate Director of Patient Safety at University Hospitals Sussex and an honorary research associate at the Department of Applied Health Research at University College London. Sam has a PhD in Patient Safety and Safety Science from UCL and has taught patient safety theory and application for the past 5 years. Sam's research now focuses on how healthcare providers can embed systems thinking and human factors theory into practice. Sam also has a background in clinical practice as an intensive care nurse and a Master of Science in Health Policy and Economics from London School of Economics.

**Samantha Warne** is Lead Editor of Patient Safety Learning's *hub,* overseeing the editorial team and responsible for developing and curating *hub* content. She is an experienced Editor, having worked on many print and online medical and scientific publications at Elsevier, the BMJ and the European Medical Group. She spent seven years working as a Website Communications

Manager at the Department of Health and more recently she was the Managing Editor at the Royal Society of Tropical Medicine & Hygiene.

**Sharon Weldon** is a Professor of Healthcare Simulation and Workforce Development. Her non-conforming application of simulation as a method has helped generate new systems of care, identified how care is perceived, tested new policies and interventions, and informed decision-making, all whilst engaging stakeholders not usually involved in such processes (patients, public, lay members). Sharon has developed surgical team training based on empirically evidenced communication models and developed innovative simulated manikins with artists and industry-partners. She has done pioneering research on sequential (care pathway-based simulations) and distributed (low cost, portable simulation equipment) simulation. This work has received funding from notable funders such as the Economic and Social Research Council, the Wellcome Trust, and the Arts and Humanities Research Council, and won several national and international awards. Her body of work in relation to simulation challenges the wider industry fixation upon concepts such as fidelity and its relevance, questioning the established knowledge and its importance in generation change and impact. She is an executive committee member for the Association for Simulated Practice in Healthcare (ASPiH) and has contributed to global white papers on simulation for patient safety. Sharon is an Associate Editor for the *International Journal of Healthcare Simulation*. More recently, she has been consulted by regulatory bodies on the use of simulation in practice and education, which has subsequently resulted in regulatory changes.

**Siri Wiig**, PhD, MSc, is Centre Director at SHARE – Centre for Resilience in Healthcare, at the University of Stavanger, Norway. The SHARE Centre is the largest research group in Norway doing research on quality and safety in healthcare. Siri is full Professor of Quality and Safety in Healthcare Systems at the Faculty of Health Sciences, UiS. Key research interests are resilience in healthcare, patient safety, quality improvement, safety investigations, user involvement, risk regulation, leadership and learning in socio-technical systems.

**Ted Baker** is Chair of the Health Services Safety Investigations Body (HSSIB), a new organisation that is tasked with undertaking systems-based investigations of safety incidents in health services in England which do not apportion blame or liability. He came to this post after an extensive career in clinical and academic medicine. He worked as a paediatric cardiologist, leading research into the establishment of magnetic resonance as a key diagnostic tool. As a clinical leader he served on the board of two large university hospital trusts as medical director and was instrumental in the inception of a new children's hospital in London. More recently he worked at the Care Quality Commission as Chief Inspector of Hospitals for England.

**Vicky Baker** works as a Senior Managers for Greater Manchester Mental Health Foundation Trust and was previously a Patient Safety lead working in the north of England. She began her career as a Registered Mental Health Nurse, working in forensic nursing in the north of England. She has since worked in a variety of clinical settings, looking to improve patient safety. She holds a Post Graduate Diploma in Human Factors for Patient Safety from the University of Stafford. She has a keen interest in learning from patient safety incidents, applying a systems and Human Factors approach to patient safety incident investigations to help explore the underlying factors to patient safety events.

**Victoria Wills** works for Gloucestershire Hospitals NHS Foundation Trust, where she has held roles in quality improvement, patient safety and Human Factors since 2015. Prior to joining the NHS, Victoria worked in the airline industry for 14 years, having joined as an apprentice at the age of 18. During that time, Victoria gained her aircraft maintenance license, a

BEng (Hons) in Air Transport Engineering and an MSc in Air Safety Management, from City University, London. Her training and engineering background led to roles within airworthiness, quality and safety, with a variety of commercial airlines across the UK and Australia. Since joining the NHS, Victoria has been instrumental in establishing the Gloucestershire Safety and Quality Improvement Academy (GSQIA), which provides quality improvement and Human Factors training to staff and provides coaching and facilitation support to a variety of quality and safety improvement projects across the Trust. Victoria has a particular interest in integrating patient safety, Human Factors and quality improvement and has, to this end, been developing approaches to support the introduction of the Patient Safety Incident Response Framework within Gloucestershire Hospitals. Victoria completed an MSc in Ergonomics and Organisational Behaviour with the University of Derby in 2022, and is a graduate member of the Chartered Institute of Ergonomics and Human Factors (CIEHF).

**Wendy Halliburton** joined the NHS in 2004 as a physiotherapist but soon found a passion for patient safety. She worked as a Patient Safety Lead across different directorates, as Patient Safety Manager and more recently as the Patient Safety Specialist. In 2023 she also took up the role of Patient Safety Lead at the Academic Health Science Network for the North East and North Cumbria (now Health Innovation). In this role she oversees the Patient Safety Collaboratives, and leads the System Safety collaborative supporting the ICB, Trusts, and independent providers who are implementing the new Patient Safety Incident Response Framework (PSIRF). Wendy undertook a Masters in Human Factors and Ergonomics at Loughborough University, graduating in 2021, and is interested in understanding systems and complexity, and exploring the use of systemic accident analysis tools for incident investigations. Her work on AcciMap and HFACS was undertaken in part as fulfilment of her Masters, and she is now supporting delivery of training in systemic accident analysis tools, including SEIPS, supporting the implementation of PSIRF within the Trust and across the region.

# Foreword

*Ted Baker*

We are living in an extraordinary time for the advancement of medical science. There have been incredible achievements in the effectiveness of the prevention and treatment of disease. Conditions once thought to be unassailable can now be treated with a high chance of a successful outcome. The United Nations estimates that average life expectancy globally in 1950 was 46.5 years; by 2019 it had risen to 72.8 years. This improvement is not only driven by economic and social factors, but also the outstanding success of modern healthcare. The developments in medical science and technology behind much of this success have been substantial and the systems to deliver healthcare have, of necessity, become increasingly complex. This complexity brings with it an increasing fragility and a risk of unintentional harm. Our understanding of this system risk and its impact on the safety of patients in our health services has undergone a transformation in recent years, but this understanding has not fully translated into practical ways that we can manage patient safety more effectively.

Traditionally, at its core, healthcare has been an interaction between an individual patient and a healthcare practitioner. For much of its history, the quality of the care was dependent on that relationship and the safety of the care relied on the diligence of the practitioner. In modern healthcare, the one-to-one patient–practitioner relationship is still central, but it no longer encompasses the totality of care. Care is provided by a system, often complex, or, in some cases, a series of interacting systems that might or might not be well coordinated around the patient's needs. Our thinking about patient safety is often still built upon the traditional view of healthcare. This conceptual barrier has stood in the way of improvements in patient safety that, in many ways, have not kept up with the advances in medical science. Indeed, the focus on safety without this understanding can and has led to a misplaced emphasis of the role of human error. Blame and recrimination when things go wrong drives a wary and defensive culture that oppresses healthcare staff and alienates their patients.

Other industries have long understood this and have transformed their approach. They have nurtured open safety cultures in which risks are reported freely without fear of retribution. They have learnt to investigate without a fixation on human fallibility, instead focusing on the system factors that create safety risks. They have embraced the best safety science to understand how systems can improve and so reduce risk. In these industries this approach has, over time, achieved spectacular improvements in safety. It is time for healthcare to catch up.

Change of this magnitude will not be easy or rapid, but we are not starting from scratch. Indeed, much work is already underway; an example being the NHS's recent far-reaching changes in reporting and investigating patient safety events and the new approaches outlined in the chapters of this book. A critical mass of expertise, crystallised in this book, has been built up over the last few years and there is an urgent desire for progress. In this book you will find guidance from those at the forefront of the patient safety movement. There are explanations of the current thinking in safety science together with practical case studies from putting it into practice. Among the topics covered is the essential work of involving patients in understanding why things go wrong and in setting priorities for safety. There have been numerous major reports on safety problems in health services over recent years and they have all had a recurrent theme; we have not listened to patients and those close to them nearly well enough. Patients' voices are vital, not just because they may have been harmed but because they have experienced safety from a different perspective. They have seen how healthcare is actually provided, not how we often imagine it is provided. If we are to improve safety, we must understand how it is experienced by patients. We must draw on their expertise and understanding. We must listen to the diversity of their views.

If we succeed, and succeed we must, improvements in patient safety will be incremental, built on consistent implementation of the best safety practice as laid out in this book. They will be cumulative, each building on those before, until eventually it is evident to all that safety has transformed and healthcare has at last come to terms with the risks inherent in its ever-increasing complexity.

# List of Abbreviations

| | |
|---|---|
| A&E | Accident and Emergency |
| AAR | After Action Review |
| AHRQ | Agency for Healthcare Research and Quality |
| AI | Appreciative Inquiry |
| AIBs | Chief Inspectors of The UK Air, Marine and Rail Accident Investigation Branches |
| ALARP | 'As low as reasonably practicable' principle |
| CA | Cardiac arrest |
| CCG | Clinical Commissioning Group |
| CIEHF | Chartered Institute of Ergonomics and Human Factors |
| CNST | Clinical Negligence Scheme for Trusts |
| CPR | Cardiopulmonary resuscitation |
| CQC | Care Quality Commission |
| CRM | Crew Resource Management |
| CUSP | Comprehensive Unit-based Safety Program |
| DSN | Diabetes Specialist Nurse |
| ED | Emergency department |
| FLO | Family Liaison Officer |
| FRAM | Functional Resonance Analysis Method |
| GHNHSFT | Gloucestershire Hospitals NHS Foundation Trust |
| GIRFT | Getting It Right First Time |
| GMC | General Medical Council |
| GSQIA | Gloucestershire Safety and Quality Improvement Academy |
| HCA | Healthcare assistant |
| HDL | High density lipoprotein |
| HFACS | Human Factors Analysis and Classification System |
| HFE | Human Factors and Ergonomics |
| HSIB | Healthcare Safety Investigation Branch |
| HSSIB | Health Services Safety Investigations Body |
| HTA | Hierarchical Task Analysis |
| ICB | Integrated Care Board |
| IMPACT | Improving Post-Event Analysis and Communication Together |
| ISA | Instantaneous Self-Assessment Method |
| I-SOG | *In Situ* Structured Observation Guide |
| LHCS | Learning healthcare system |
| MDT | Multidisciplinary team |
| M&M | Mortality and morbidity |
| MNSI | Maternity and Newborn Safety Investigations |

| | |
|---|---|
| MoU | Memorandum of Understanding |
| NEWS2 | National Early Warning Score |
| NHS | National Health Service |
| NIHR | National Institute for Health and Care Research |
| NMC | Nursing and Midwifery Council |
| NPCC | National Police Chiefs' Council |
| NPIA | National Policing Improvement Agency |
| NTC | National Training Centre |
| OD | Once Daily |
| OECD | Organisation for Economic Co-Operation and Development |
| OOH | Out of Hours |
| PALS | Patient Advice and Liaison Service |
| PDA | Patent ductus arteriosus |
| PDSA | Plan, Do, Study, Act |
| PEARLS | Promoting Excellence and Reflective Learning in Simulation (PEARLS) |
| PFLO | Patient and Family Liaison Officer |
| PHSO | Parliamentary and Health Service Ombudsman |
| PIF | Performance influencing factor |
| PMRT | Perinatal Mortality Review Tools |
| PPE | Personal protective equipment |
| PPH | Post-partum haemorrhage |
| PSII | Patient safety incident investigation |
| PSIRF | Patient Safety Incident Response Framework |
| PSIRP | Patient Safety Incident Response Plan |
| PSMN | Patient Safety Management Network |
| PSRC | Patient Safety Research Collaboration |
| QI | Quality Improvement |
| RCA | Root cause analysis |
| Rx | Prescription |
| SAA | Systemic accident analysis |
| SBI | Seven simulation-based 'Is' |
| SEIPS | System Engineering Initiative for Patient Safety |
| SI | Serious Incident |
| SIF | Serious Incident Framework |
| SMART | Specific, Measurable, Achievable, Realistic and Timely |
| SOP | Standard operating procedure |
| SPO | Structure-process-outcomes |
| STAMP | Systems-Theoretic Accident Model and Processes |
| SWOT | Strengths, Weaknesses, Opportunities and Threats |
| TT | Testicular Torsion |
| UK | United Kingdom |
| US | United States |
| WHO | World Health Organization |
| WT3 | Walk-Through-Talk-Through |

# CHAPTER 1

# Introduction

*Claire Cox, Jordan Nicholls and Helen Hughes*

Modern healthcare is complex. There are a range of different ways in which unintended avoidable harm can occur, with millions of patients harmed or dying each year across the world because of this. In the United Kingdom (UK), the National Health Service (NHS) pre-Covid-19 estimate was that there were around 11,000 avoidable deaths annually due to safety concerns, with thousands more seriously harmed (NHS England and NHS Improvement, 2019).

Patient safety as a discipline has emerged in response to this and the evolving intricacy of healthcare. It can be defined as:

'A framework of organized activities that creates cultures, processes, procedures, behaviours, technologies and environments in health care that consistently and sustainably lower risks, reduce the occurrence of avoidable harm, make errors less likely and reduce the impact of harm when it does occur.' (WHO, 2021)

A key feature of this is collecting data on patient safety events and using these insights and experiences to improve our understanding of why such incidents occur and to help inform solutions to prevent their recurrence.

## Patient Safety in the NHS

During the 1980s and 1990s there was an increasing awareness of the impact of avoidable harm in healthcare, marked by the publication in 1999 of the seminal Institute of Medicine report, *To Err is Human*. This set out that the level of hospital deaths as a result of avoidable harm in the United States of America (US) could be as high as 98,000 per year (Institute of Medicine, 1999). At around the same time in the UK, the Chief Medical Officer published *An Organisation with a Memory*, a report focused on learning from adverse events in the NHS. This highlighted the need for significant improvements to the health system's approach to patient safety, noting that 'the NHS is failing to learn from the things that go wrong and has no system to put this right' (Department of Health, 2000).

Following the publication of *An Organisation with a Memory*, patient safety as a concept has increasingly been in the mainstream of healthcare in the UK. There has been a growing consciousness of the need to better understand the causes of unsafe care and the action needed to reduce harm, coupled with a range of new roles, programmes and initiatives created to this end. However, despite the hard work of many people involved in the industry, avoidable harm has continued to persist at high levels.

There have been a wide range of discussions about the reasons for the persistence of harm. Some have focused on the way we think about and approach improving safety in healthcare and the need to balance between Safety-I and Safety-II approaches (Hollnagel and Wears, 2015), which we consider in greater detail in Chapter 5. Others have looked at what is needed to tackle the implementation gap between what we know improves patient safety and what is done in practice (Woodward, 2016) and the need to address the complex systemic causes that underpin avoidable harm (Patient Safety Learning, 2019).

In the NHS itself, the heart of the current approach to improving patient safety is the *NHS Patient Safety Strategy*. Published in July 2019, this strategy sets out how the NHS should work towards its safety vision 'to continuously improve patient safety' (NHS England and NHS Improvement, 2019). It sets out three strategic aims to help build a patient safety culture and patient safety system to achieve this: insight, involvement and improvement.

The 'insight' strategy focuses on how best the health system can draw intelligence from multiple sources of patient safety information. It identifies a key element of this as a new Patient Safety Incident Response Framework (PSIRF), which:

> '... sets out the NHS's approach to developing and maintaining effective systems and processes for responding to patient safety incidents for the purpose of learning and improving patient safety' (NHS England, 2022a).

NHS England states that the four key aims of PSIRF are:

1. Compassionate engagement and involvement of those affected by patient safety incidents.
2. Application of a range of system-based approaches to learning from patient safety incidents.
3. Considered and proportionate responses to patient safety incidents.
4. Supportive oversight focused on strengthening response system functioning and improvement. (NHS England, 2022a)

This new framework has given rise to new-found opportunities and freedom of investigation and incident management. However, its proposals also represent a significant shift in approach to incident investigation, with these new approaches to learning, action and improvement requiring significant training and, in some cases, a radical change in mindset. To ensure that NHS organisations apply these new approaches and tools, guidance has been issued (NHS England, 2022b), including advice on the culture change needed with a focus on learning and improvement together with PSIRF training for all staff.

## Practical Tools for Patient Safety

*Patient Safety: Emerging Applications of Safety Science*, is written *by* people working in patient safety management *for* patient safety management people. It explores the theory of safety and translates this into practice using a case study approach. Although the trigger for this book is the implementation of PSIRF, the reasons behind this book and the challenges faced across the healthcare system are inherently worldwide.

The impetus for this book comes from discussions and growth of the Patient Safety Management Network (PSMN). The PSMN is an informal voluntary network of patient safety professionals, created by and for patient safety managers and hosted on the charity Patient Safety Learning's online platform, *the hub*. Established in 2021, the PSMN has become a key forum for discussion about the implementation of PSIRF. It is a safe space for regular discussions about the new system-based approaches to investigations outlined in PSIRF and provides a valuable resource and place to share experiences and good practice (Cox, 2021). Many of the case studies in this book come from members of the PSMN. The Network has grown rapidly and the membership is expanding (Cox, 2023), demonstrating that there is a clear appetite and interest from patient safety professionals to share learning about new approaches to patient safety. The PSMN model of collaboration, engagement and knowledge sharing has inspired the creation of other patient safety focused communities of interest, including the Patient Safety Partners Network, the National Safety Standards for Invasive Procedures (NatSSIPs) Network, all supported by Patient Safety Learning.

*Patient Safety: Emerging Applications of Safety Science* is filled with good-practice case studies from the frontline that can be adapted by others to use in their organisations. In '*Mind the implementation gap*', Patient Safety Learning (2022) discussed the difference between what we know improves patient safety and what is done in practice and highlights the key reason for this is the implementation gap. In this book we highlight the issues with dissemination of these tools and methodologies; 'work as imagined' compared with 'work as done'. Chapter 3 considers the practical application of the System Engineering Initiative for Patient Safety (SEIPS) in healthcare, a model used in many other industries and now being applied in healthcare along new investigative tools promoted as part of PSIRF.

## Engagement with Patients and Families

The importance of patient engagement in improving health outcomes, reducing harm and enhancing trust in health systems is increasingly being recognised both in the UK and across the world (WHO, 2023a). 'Engaging patients for patient safety' was the theme of World Patient Safety Day 2023 (WHO, 2023b), in recognition of the crucial role patients, families and caregivers play in the safety of healthcare. For decades safety investigations and reports have highlighted failures to listen to and involve patients in their care and when harm has occurred. Patient Safety Learning identified patient engagement as one of the six foundations of safer care in their report, *A Blueprint for Action* (Patient Safety Learning, 2019). Improving and increasing patient and family engagement is also one of the seven strategic objectives of the World Health Organization (WHO) Global Patient Safety Action Plan (WHO, 2021).

We have learned through the PSMN meetings that across some organisations there is a huge gap in family liaison and support when a patient is harmed, and that extends to PSIRF. Patients who have been harmed or people who have lost a loved one to avoidable harm are likely to have different reasons for wanting an investigation. Without adequate communication and support, investigations can be very distressing for patients and their families. How can we engage with patients and families without compounding the harm they have already experienced? Working and supporting patients who have been harmed and their loved ones can sometimes be challenging. We need to make sure we're communicating well and meet the needs of patients and families. We also need to make sure our staff are supported with guidance, advice and have the right skills.

*Patient Safety: Emerging Applications of Safety Science* explores the key reasons why patient and family engagement following patient safety incidents is important, introducing the concept of 'compounded harm' and explores some of the ways we can learn and improve through the case studies.

## Proactive Safety within Healthcare

We see this book as the 'discovery' phase of the journey. These methodologies are well established in other industries, and with the introduction of PSIRF we now have the opportunity to embrace and strengthen our approach to healthcare safety.

By including real life examples from the frontline, this book highlights the gaps between the theory and application and identifies where further resources are needed, so we can not only learn from patient safety incidents but also learn how to practice proactive safety within healthcare.

It is also important not to lose sight of the wider patient safety context. Avoidable harm in healthcare is driven by a range of complex systemic causes that underpin this. To tackle these causes requires a broader transformation in our approach to patient safety, placing this as a core purpose of health and care. Improving our approach to learning and investigation is one part of this that needs to be supported by strong patient safety leadership and governance arrangements operating within organisational cultures that encourage and support learning for patient safety.

# References

Cox, C. (2021). *Patient Safety Management Network — the time is now*. Patient Safety Learning: *the hub*. www.pslhub.org/learn/improving-patient-safety/patient-safety-management-network-the-time-is-now-25-october-2021-r5412/.

Cox, C. (2023). *The voices of the patient safety frontline — the Patient Safety Management Network two years on*. Patient Safety Learning: *the hub*. https://www.pslhub.org/learn/professionalising-patient-safety/the-voices-of-the-patient-safety-frontline-the-patient-safety-management-network-two-years-on-r9894/.

Department of Health (2000). *An organisation with a memory*. https://www.sciencedirect.com/science/article/pii/S147021182403879X?via%3Dihub/.

Hollnagel, E. and Wears, R.L. (2015). *From Safety-I to Safety-II: A White Paper*. https://www.england.nhs.uk/signuptosafety/wp-content/uploads/sites/16/2015/10/safety-1-safety-2-whte-papr.pdf.

Institute of Medicine (1999). *To Err is Human: Building a Safe Health System*. www.ncbi.nlm.nih.gov/books/NBK225182/.

NHS England (2022a). *Patient Safety Incident Response Framework*. https://www.england.nhs.uk/patient-safety/patient-safety-insight/incident-response-framework/.

NHS England (2022b). *Patient Safety Incident Response Framework and supporting guidance*. www.england.nhs.uk/publication/patient-safety-incident-response-framework-and-supporting-guidance/.

NHS England and NHS Improvement (2019). *The NHS Patient Safety Strategy*. www.england.nhs.uk/patient-safety/the-nhs-patient-safety-strategy/.

Patient Safety Learning (2019). *The Patient-Safe Future: A Blueprint for Action*. https://d2z1laakrytay6.cloudfront.net/content/A-Blueprint-for-Action-240619.pdf.

WHO (2021). *Global Patient Safety Action Plan 2021–2030*. https://www.who.int/publications/i/item/9789240032705.

WHO (2023a). *Engaging Patients for Patient Safety: Advocacy Brief*. https://iris.who.int/bitstream/handle/10665/375011/9789240081987-eng.pdf.

WHO (2023b). *World Patient Safety Day 2023. Engaging Patients for Patient Safety*. www.who.int/news-room/events/detail/2023/09/17/default-calendar/world-patient-safety-day-2023--engaging-patients-for-patient-safety.

Woodward (2016). *Patient Safety: closing the implementation gap*. www.kingsfund.org.uk/blog/2016/08/patient-safety-closing-implementation-gap.

CHAPTER 2

# The Theory of Change Management and its Application in Quality and Safety

*Julie Storr*

## Summary

This chapter starts with a brief recap on some of the key historical milestones in the field of change management and patient safety that have influenced and continue to frame current thinking. It then explores numerous dominant change theories, both within and outside of the healthcare context, focusing on common themes emerging from the research. Drawing on the research, the chapter maps a number of the common barriers and challenges and considers potential mitigations. The chapter concludes with an exploration of how change management principles can be optimally applied to the field of patient safety.

## Background

'If you leave a thing alone you leave it to a torrent of change.'

G.K. Chesterton (Ratcliffe, 2016)

The history of healthcare is replete with change initiatives, from small-scale interventions at the level of an individual unit, through to massive transformational change across entire health systems, sometimes spanning continents. Indeed, change management has been at the centre of efforts to bring about the step change required to enhance the safety and quality of healthcare. Yet change failure in this context has been described as omnipresent, ranging from small technical errors within new systems, processes or technologies, through to breakdowns and large-scale disaster (Schwarz *et al.*, 2021).

Large-scale patient safety disasters in many countries have driven efforts to improve patient safety. As far back as the late 1980s, staff concerns over the quality of paediatric cardiac surgery in the UK (Bristol) resulted in a national investigation and report (Kennedy, 2001) that catalysed change in patient safety and quality. As Vincent (2010) recalls, the then editor of the *British Medical Journal* wrote an editorial 'All changed, changed utterly, British Medicine will be transformed by the Bristol case' (Smith, 1998). This case catalysed a transformation and achieved 'the remarkable feat of bringing positive, forward-looking change from disaster and tragedy' (Vincent, 2010). A similar pattern emerged in a number of other countries around the same time, in particular the US (Kohn *et al.*, 1999).

In the intervening years, patient safety has evolved into a mature global movement, recognised at the highest level as fundamental to the quality of healthcare. There is currently a WHO global action plan that runs through to 2030, supported by every country of the world (WHO, 2021). This plan highlights the importance of fully understanding the process of change and utilising the established body of knowledge on improvement science to achieve the desired outcome of zero avoidable harm. WHO highlight the need to work closely with leaders, managers, professional staff and patient representatives in health facilities and clinical services, and nurture centres of excellence, learn from them and scale up proven best practices.

Hughes (2023) lists seven underlying system issues that contribute to avoidable harm remaining an unsolved problem in the twenty-first century: (i) safety is one of many strategic priorities faced by healthcare leaders; (ii) there are few safety standards and defining what 'good patient safety' looks like is problematic; (iii) patient safety is seldom hardwired into the development of healthcare procedures, processes, products and systems; (iv) organisational cultures within healthcare continue to be predominantly blame focused; (v) patient centredness remains elusive; (vi) patient safety leadership is difficult to achieve and models for leadership and governance for patient safety are largely lacking; and (vii) where effective solutions do exist, there is too often a lack of means by which these are shared more widely. Tackling these requires a robust understanding of change management theory, models and tools. Ramanujam et al. (2005) suggest that patient safety initiatives can succeed only to the extent to which healthcare organisations recognise the need for and develop the means to implement the necessary organisational changes. Historically, healthcare has been criticised for not devoting enough attention to the theory of change management (Noble et al., 2011).

# The Theory Behind Change Management

## Change Management Outside of Healthcare

The body of knowledge on change management that healthcare has drawn on has some of its origins in the field of manufacturing, where, in an effort to improve product quality, there was a recognition of the need to transition from 'managing by imposing control' to 'managing by eliciting commitment' (Ramanujam et al., 2005). Barrow et al. (2022) summarise four of the classic change management theories that have been studied to determine their relevance to healthcare: Lewin's three-step process for ensuring successful change; Lippitt's seven phases; Kotter's eight-step Change Model; and Rogers' diffusion of innovation theory (Box 2.1).

---

**BOX 2.1**    Four Dominant Change Theories According to Barrow et al. (2022)

### Lewin's Planned Change Theory

1. Unfreezing (understanding change is needed).
2. Moving (the process of initiating change).
3. Refreezing (establishing a new status quo).

### Lippitt's Phases of Change Theory

1. Becoming more aware of the need for change.
2. Developing a relationship between the system and change agent.
3. Defining a change problem.
4. Setting change goals and action plans for achievement.
5. Implementing the change.
6. Staff acceptance of the change — stabilisation.
7. Redefining the relationship of the change agent with the system.

## Kotter's Eight-Step Change Model
1. Creating a sense of urgency for change.
2. Forming a guiding change team.
3. Creating a vision and plan for change.
4. Communicating the change vision and plan with stakeholders.
5. Removing change barriers.
6. Providing short-term wins.
7. Building on the change.
8. Making the change stick in the culture.

## Rogers' Diffusion of Innovation Theory
1. Knowledge (education and communication to expose staff to the change).
2. Persuasion (use of change champions to pique staff interest; peers persuading peers).
3. Decision (staff decide whether to accept or reject the change).
4. Implementation (putting new processes into practice).
5. Confirmation (staff recognise the value and benefits of the change and continue to use changed processes).

Common across each is an attempt to describe key activities required in the process of moving from an undesirable to a desirable state. Phillips *et al.* (2023) consider the dichotomy posed by looking at change through an academic versus a practical lens. They suggest that academics tend to use terms such as models, theories and concepts, whereas practitioners use tools and techniques. The authors acknowledge that there is no one-size-fits-all approach, due in part to the chaotic nature of change, but that many models and frameworks consist of similar change management strategies. In a survey of change managers, they draw out five common change management strategies that mirror the theories presented in Box 2.1: (i) communicate about the change; (ii) involve stakeholders at all levels of the organisation; (iii) focus on organisational culture; (iv) consider the organisation's mission and vision; and (v) provide encouragement and incentives to change.

## Change Management within the Healthcare System

Over a decade ago, Noble and colleagues posited the question: what has change management in industry got to do with improving patient safety? (Noble *et al.*, 2011). In their paper the authors presented an analysis of the literature on change to suggest how this may inform patient safety, acknowledging the seminal change model of Kotter, and concluded that Kotter's model has potential to be adapted for improving patient safety. Kotter's steps, or variations thereof, has been increasingly used within the context of healthcare (Burden, 2016; Karimi *et al.*, 2022). Karimi *et al.* also identified the importance of considering resistance to change and potential solutions to resistance as important factors when preparing for change. The criticality of leadership is highlighted. This will become a recurring theme in this chapter. The authors discuss the need to consider context and situation in relation to the use of change management strategies. From their review, a common set of activities that must be considered are listed, including assessing the need and readiness for change, creating project management and responsive teams or stakeholder committees, a participatory approach, removal of obstacles, and the importance of soliciting regular feedback.

During recent decades, the use of Appreciative Inquiry (AI) has been documented in healthcare change management initiatives (Watkins *et al.*, 2000) and has been described as a motivational, organisational change intervention, which can be used to improve the quality and safety of healthcare (Merriel *et al.*, 2022). Instead of focusing on problems, AI is a problem-solving approach that turns conventional thinking on its head by encouraging members of an organisation to focus on discovering what is working well and envisioning a future where this becomes the norm (Coghlan *et al.*, 2003). In his work moving from Safety-I to Safety-II, Hollnagel *et al.* (2015) has pioneered this notion of learning from what goes right and building systems to support sharing of learning across healthcare. Participants in the AI process discuss what resources and activities are needed to bring about the desired future and they then implement the desired changes. Coghlan and colleagues consider one of the unique selling points of AI to be the engagement and inspiration it engenders in participants for the change. Although Merriel and colleagues found minimal empirical evidence to support the effectiveness of AI in improving healthcare, they concluded that the qualitative and observational evidence suggests it may have a positive impact on clinical care, leading to improved patient and organisational outcomes.

Porritt *et al.* (2020), in their *Handbook for Evidence Implementation*, provide guidance to health professionals, researchers and public health practitioners planning to implement evidence into their setting. The handbook states that successful implementation in healthcare is all about change management. The authors highlight the importance of considering the human as well as the technical resources needed to complete any implementation project. They state that such projects require a team of people to engage with others and enact a process of change and change management and recommend that this team is established well before confirmation of the project topic, scope and direction to ensure the project is feasible and will be accepted across the organisation. They go on to state that a dominant theme across all literature about change management, and therefore implementation science, is the acknowledgement that leadership support is essential — particularly when it comes to large, complex organisations such as hospitals.

The concept of a learning healthcare system (LHCS) has also come to the fore in recent years and is of relevance in the context of healthcare change management. *Crossing the Global Quality Chasm: Improving Health Care Worldwide* (National Academies of Sciences, 2018) describe the role that LHCSs can play in establishing a culture of continual learning. An LHCS is described as an organisation that uses continuous cycles of learning and reflection to inspire growth and development, involving all stakeholders — staff, managers, executives, clinicians, patients, communities and others. LHCSs are concerned with transforming clinical care and better aligning people, processes and technology through routinising continuous, rapid and systematic evidence generation into medical practice (Smoyer *et al.*, 2016). LHCSs follow a cycle of gathering data, analysing and making sense of the data, and feeding the findings back into practice to support productive change. This cycle is similar to the Plan, Do, Study, Act (PDSA) cycle used widely in quality improvement (QI) (Varkey *et al.*, 2011). In Chapter 3 on the Systems Engineering Initiative for Patient Safety (SEIPS), case study 2 illustrates the value of PDSA in testing and assessing change ideas. An LHCS is described in the 'Crossing the global quality chasm' report as a 'change machine', seeking to close the gap between knowledge and action and quicken the pace of change, supporting the rapid testing of best practices and lessons and their incorporation into routine clinical practice (IOM, 2011). Similar to AI, LHCSs seek to identify failures and reduce them to an irreducible minimum, so employing elements of the Safety-II approach toward resilient healthcare. The focus, again, is on understanding what makes things go right in a complex, non-linear healthcare system. The report emphasises that an LHCS can engage with clinicians and all providers to identify and promote the characteristics and circumstances that lead to good care, and then make that information available to others to extend the network of learning and bring about positive change.

## Improving the Safety of Care Delivery — A Universal Challenge

The challenge of patient safety has been described as intertwined with, and almost indistinguishable from, the challenge of organisational change (Ramanujam et al., 2005). Twenty years on from the birth of the modern patient safety movement, patients continue to be harmed, lessons continue to fail to be learned and there remains a need for system-wide change and a renewed focus on turning the lessons learned when things go wrong into practical change (Patient Safety Learning, 2019).

Improving and sustaining quality and safety in healthcare is a challenge for reasons touched on in the previous section. The challenges posed by the complexity of the healthcare system itself and its many networks, each with their own people, processes and cultures, cannot be understated (Vincent, 2010). Furthermore, the challenge of patient safety is not solely a clinical one, but also organisational (Ramanujam et al., 2005). To this end, success is predicated on the use of change management principles in the design and execution of patient safety initiatives. In particular there is a need to institutionalise change through capacitating the workforce and ensuring continuous learning.

These challenges are an Achilles heel in the journey to safer care and influence the slow translation of evidence of effectiveness into routine practice — described as the 'know-do' gap, the gap between what is known to be effective care ('know') and what is routinely performed by providers ('do') to close the gap (WHO 2018a, WHO 2021). WHO, Organisation for Economic Co-operation and Development (OECD) and World Bank in their landmark report on delivering quality health services (WHO, 2018a) call for multimodal changes in clinical practice at every level of a health system, 'from the individual encounter between the patient and the health care worker to the redesign of health care delivery'. Such a multimodal approach acknowledges the behavioural dimension of the changes required to improve quality and safety, and the authors emphasise harm reduction to patients as a key objective. However, the report goes on to state that programmes that focus only on provider behaviour fail to recognise the importance of the wider environment of healthcare in supporting or obstructing best practice. The example of antibiotic prescribing is used to illustrate the complexity of the changes required, that include the need to acknowledge the influence of practice guidelines, performance feedback, peer review, training and supervision, financial incentives, availability of a sufficient variety of antibiotics and patient expectation.

Such barriers have also been highlighted by other authors. Shojania et al. (2005) in a review of evidence-based QI and the barriers faced when translating evidence to practice found incentives (or lack of) including, but not solely, financial incentives; structural barriers; peer group behaviour; professional knowledge; attitudes and beliefs; and finally patient factors. There is a strong but not exclusive behavioural component to such barriers. Taitz et al. (2011) also determined that physician lack of time, the institutional culture, physicians' desire for autonomy, insufficient training and general lack of QI skills among improvers were key barriers. In a study by the Health Foundation (Davies et al., 2007), health professionals in the UK self-identified five barriers to change that included lack of time; lack of resources; high workload, inadequate managerial support and inadequate access to the necessary skills to implement improvement (therapists only); staff shortages, lack of authority and the need for active consultant support and difficulties reconciling research evidence with practice reality (nurses only); and finally a wide range of disparate barriers cited by physicians that included incompatible computer systems, lack of administrative support and individual fears of being undermined by assessment and criticism. This study then considered the facilitators that directly addressed each of the barriers listed with a strong emphasis on the important role that leadership plays, including opinion leaders, the power of effective team training, multidisciplinary working, pay for performance and financial incentives. These barriers were further reinforced in a policy analysis by Allcock *et al.* (2015) who identified barriers to change in four areas: recognition of the need to change; having the motivation to change; headspace to make change happen; and the capability to execute change.

In a review of the academic literature and the UK Health Foundation's QI programmes, Dixon-Woods *et al.* (2012) identified ten challenges to QI programme implementation falling under four broad themes: design and planning; organisational and institutional contexts; professions and leadership; and sustainability and spread and unintended consequences. In considering the bridging of the theory and practice of change management, Table 2.1 maps the challenges outlined by Dixon-Woods and colleagues against the potential barriers to change, informed by the work of Kotter (2007). This highlights some interesting commonalities and helps to frame a number of potential mitigation strategies, particularly drawing on the Dixon-Woods *et al.* report, for the consideration of those embarking on a change project. The reader is invited to consider their own mitigations, framed by their local context and culture.

**Table 2.1** Mapping Change Barriers, Challenges and Mitigations (informed by Kotter and Dixon-Woods *et al.*)

| Potential Barrier (informed by Kotter, 2007) | Key Challenge (adapted from Dixon-Woods *et al.*, 2012) | Illustrative Potential Mitigations |
|---|---|---|
| Not establishing a great enough sense of urgency for the change | Lack of leadership | • High-level leadership from the outset e.g. CEO leads the change from day one<br>• Engagement of senior leaders from across different professional groups |
| Not creating a powerful enough guiding coalition | Inability to convince people that the solution chosen is the right one | • Creation of small leadership teams who commit to take the necessary action needed to implement change |
| Lacking a vision | An organisational context, culture and capacity not fit for purpose | • Use multiple communication channels to sell the vision |
| Under-communicating the vision by a factor of 10 | Failure to convince people that there is a problem | • Radical review and enhancement of all existing communication channels<br>• Consider campaign fatigue<br>• Develop key messages for leaders to use<br>• Use hard (local) data to sell the problem |
| Not removing obstacles to the new vision | Tribalism and lack of staff engagement | • Empower and engage staff<br>• Agree roles and responsibilities and protect staff time for the change |
| Not systematically planning for and creating short term wins | Insufficient data systems and an imbalance between carrots and sticks | • Don't underestimate the intrinsic motivations of staff for quality improvement<br>• Actively seek out small successes and use all communication channels to publicise<br>• Consider external support<br>• Use 'sticks' to encourage change judiciously |

| Potential Barrier (informed by Kotter, 2007) | Key Challenge (adapted from Dixon-Woods et al., 2012) | Illustrative Potential Mitigations |
|---|---|---|
| Declaring victory too soon | Excess ambitions and failure to consider the side effects of change | • Celebrate progress and achievement<br>• Focus on the long-term<br>• Review vulnerabilities to explore extent of success<br>• Be aware of unintended consequences |
| Not anchoring changes in the corporate culture | Inability to secure sustainability | • Constantly communicate the approach, successes and changes to processes and performance using all available channels<br>• Routinise successful outcomes into standards, guidelines and procedures |

The psychological impact of organisational change on employees is another challenge encountered when introducing change in healthcare, with studies documenting that high rates of change do affect health and well-being (Day et al., 2017). Having the opportunity to influence the change, being prepared for the change and valuing the change can help to mitigate this psychological impact. In addition, Ramanujam et al. (2005) consider the costs of mismanaging change that extend beyond the failure of the patient safety initiative itself, often extending to a sceptical workforce with lower buy-in to future patient safety initiatives.

# Examples of Change Management and Patient Safety in a Complex System

## The Importance of Leadership

It is clear that leadership is a fundamental feature of successful change management. Miller (2001) emphasises the centrality of strong and committed leadership to successful major change. According to Miller, successful change leaders build high levels of commitment, are disciplined, choose the right implementation framework and are systematic and relentless in its execution. As evidenced in Table 2.1, Dixon-Woods et al. (2012) further emphasise the importance of engaging respected individuals to play a vital role in encouraging colleagues across different professions to buy in to any improvement and suggest that the key factor for success may lie in a 'quieter' leadership focused on collaboration. In their seven success factors for 'good change' (Allcock et al., 2015), leadership either directly or indirectly transcends most of the list, which includes committed and respected leadership that engages staff; a culture hospitable to, and supportive of, change; and enabling an environment which supports and drives the change and resources and support for the change.

## Change, Implementation and Improvement

Change and improvement are often used interchangeably in the literature. For example, Allcock et al. use continuous improvement to describe small-scale incremental changes — which can, over time, produce significantly different services, and use the term 'transformation' to describe large-scale change across an organisation or multiple organisations. Hughes (2008) presents a synthesis of the literature on QI and its relevance to patient safety, in which QI is defined as systematic, data-guided activities designed to bring about immediate improvement in healthcare delivery in particular settings to address identified gaps. QI and a familiar approach involves use of the PDSA model. PDSA cycles are concerned with establishing the causal relationship between changes in processes (specifically behaviours and capabilities) and outcomes. Three questions are initially asked, in any order: (i) what are we trying to accomplish?; (ii) how will we know that a change is an improvement?; and (iii) what change can we make that will result in improvement? (WHO, 2018b). Other quality improvement tools include six sigma, failure modes and effects analysis and root cause analysis (RCA) to name but a few (Hughes, 2008).

Established methods of quality improvement can be used to design and redesign systems and processes to improve patient safety (WHO, 2021). These models of change, stemming from the field of improvement science, provide a structured approach to changing practices and processes.

## Application of Change Management Principles to Patient Safety

A number of patient safety improvement initiatives across different levels of the health system have used change management approaches. Hughes (2023) emphasises the importance of understanding the gap between 'work as imagined' and 'work as done' because this is often where patient safety initiatives and products can come undone. Hughes goes on to state that in seeking to improve patient safety and reduce avoidable harm, it is vital to engage with how work takes place on the ground and not solely rely on the idea of how it should take place. With this in mind, this chapter concludes with a real-world example of the integration of change management principles within efforts to improve patient safety: the Comprehensive Unit-based Safety Program (CUSP). CUSP is a framework, developed by patient safety researchers at the Johns Hopkins Hospital in the US, with the aim of improving safety culture and guiding organisations to learn from mistakes (Weaver *et al.*, 2015). CUSP has been used in many countries to address multiple vulnerabilities across all levels of a healthcare organisation and to identify and eliminate patient safety hazards (Weaver *et al.*, 2013). Inter-related organisational vulnerabilities put at risk an organisation's capacity to achieve excellence in the area of safety and quality. Dixon-Woods *et al.* (2011) provide a possible explanation for the persistence of such vulnerabilities in terms of the 'Cargo Cult of QI', whereby initiatives are implemented without a full understanding of what they involve and how they work, resulting in the superficial outer appearance but not the mechanisms that produce the desired outcomes.

The CUSP approach and its set of interventions aim to mitigate Cargo Cult thinking and address what Pronovost (2011) described as the recalcitrant adaptive challenges facing those wanting to improve patient safety and quality. CUSP is built around Kotter's eight steps and consists of five steps (Johns Hopkins Medicine, 2015). It has been validated in the context of improving safety culture and reducing healthcare-associated infection in the intensive care unit (Berenholtz *et al.*, 2014) and the surgical setting (Timmel *et al.*, 2010), reducing mortality (Lipitz-Snyderman *et al.*, 2011), and within long-term care its use has been demonstrated in the context of preventing healthcare associated infection (AHRQ, 2015).

The five steps centre on: (i) education of staff on the science of safety; (ii) engagement of staff to identify defects; (iii) involvement of executives; (iv) learning from defects; and (v) implementing tools for improvement. CUSP is predicated on the idea that many healthcare organisations possess all the capability, processes and solutions to address the technical challenges they face in theory. What CUSP offers is a strategy to address the adaptive challenges; the problems not amenable to authoritative expertise or guidelines, the ones that require experiments, new discoveries and adjustments, including changing attitudes, values and behaviours. CUSP is further underpinned by behavioural science theories and also influenced by the diffusion of innovation theory (Pronovost *et al.*, 2008).

Each of the five steps is designed to empower the workforce to assume responsibility for safety in their environment. Preceding the five steps the approach requires the establishment of an inter-disciplinary safety team that drives improvement (Johns Hopkins Medicine, 2015). This pre-implementation action aims to galvanise individuals and teams and lay the foundations for success. These teams will act as the driving force for improvement and should represent all the disciplines working on a unit, including nurses, physicians, pharmacists and support staff, reflecting the key role of all workers in safety. During this on-boarding phase, the commitment of senior executives takes place. It is during this phase that measurement and improvement data are also gathered that will be used throughout the intervention, including a culture assessment. Using all the information gathered during steps 1–4, safety team members highlight priorities for improvement action. The CUSP approach recommends the use of established quality improvement tools and suggests selecting three improvements per year. A number of tools are recommended for universal application, including learning from defects, shadowing another profession, observing rounds and a culture debriefing tool. Each of the improvements has an associated metric. The core CUSP Toolkit is available via the Agency for Healthcare Research and Quality (AHRQ).

Through this systematic process of what has been termed the Four Es — engagement, education, execution and evaluation — Pronovost and colleagues outline how using such an approach targets the different levels of the workforce that need to be targeted for successful change: executive leaders, team leaders and frontline workers. At each level a number of questions are posed, the answers to which guide the overall improvement, inspire change and motivate the organisation as a collective to safer practices (Box 2.2).

### BOX 2.2 Questions to Guide Improvement

#### Executive Level
- What is the role of the leader in creating a better, safer organisation aligned with its current vision and values?
- What knowledge gaps exist?
- Is there a business case for safety?
- Are the board of directors engaged?
- Are monitoring strategies in place?

#### Team Leader Level
- What is the precise role of the team leader in creating safety units and winning hearts and minds?

#### Individual Workforce Level
- Do workers have self-efficacy in relation to the change?
- Do workers believe in their role in patient safety?

As executive leaders will ultimately drive the improvement, their task is to consider the actions needed to make the change a reality, including a focus on necessary skills and resources. Team leaders are critical in driving the implementation of bespoke improvement. As improvement progresses toward implementation of action plans, individual workers need to be directed and their commitment secured to the operational reality of improvement. At each of the three levels, evaluation is a key feature. Being able to demonstrate that an improvement has been made is critical to executive leaders. Team leaders will focus on ensuring systems are in place to demonstrate real-time learning and improvement, taking account of current vulnerabilities.

The Four Es has subsequently been incorporated within international implementation manuals focused on improvement interventions for the reduction of surgical site infection (WHO, 2018c). The similarities and relationship between the Four Es' approach and WHO's multimodal improvement strategy (Allegranzi et al., 2013), another strategy to support change in healthcare, was demonstrated. Both approaches share a common focus in that they point out 'how' improvement programmes can be organised to successfully support and enable the implementation of technical prevention measures and bring about behavioural and structural change within complex healthcare environments. A more recent illustration of the use of the CUSP approach and its impact by Gu et al. (2021) focused on adverse events associated with the intrahospital transfer of patients with critical diseases. The authors explored the effect of applying CUSP and the paper concluded that implementation of CUSP can significantly shorten the in-hospital transfer time, improve the attitude of medical staff towards safety, reduce the occurrence rate of adverse events and improve the satisfaction of patients' relatives to the transfer process.

## A Practical Framework for Change Management — the NHS Change Model

The English NHS developed the Change Model, a practical framework that provides the end user with ideas, prompts, tools and resources that can be tailored to local contexts. The Change Model has eight components which set out the elements that should be considered when planning and implementing change (Box 2.3).

---

**BOX 2.3    Eight Components of the Change Model**

1. Our shared purpose — the starting point
2. Spread and adoption
3. Improvement tools
4. Project and performance management
5. Measurement
6. System drivers
7. Motivate and mobilise
8. Leadership by all

---

The Change Model Guide, action planning templates and gap analysis tools together with key questions to guide the process of change, can be accessed here: www.england.nhs.uk/gp/national-general-practice-improvement-programme/change-model/.

## Conclusion

A number of the case studies presented in the following chapters bring to life the human element of change; change is about people, both those on the front line and those who lead. For example, in Chapter 6, case study 1 highlights how the use of After Action Reviews (AARs) helped to empower staff to be part of the identified change. In Chapter 8, Jayne Wheway and Patrick Waterson present the six steps involved in constructing an AcciMap, an accident investigation tool used extensively in safety critical industries worldwide. Step 6 involves a 'team check and validation' of the proposed changes. This contributes to a shared understanding, a reduction of blame and provides a place for interactive exploration for those with the role to create change.

Together with the available literature it is clear that staff working in health and care are motivated by a vision of safe care and better ways to deliver quality (Dougall *et al.*, 2018). Frontline staff are critical in achieving safer care; however, they must be supported by organisational leaders to bring about the changes needed for quality care (Ham *et al.*, 2016).

Change management, QI and patient safety are somewhat intertwined within the literature. This chapter highlights that change management has been widely studied within the social sciences outside of a healthcare context and there is much to learn from this. Understanding change theory appears central to choosing the most appropriate change management strategy and in addressing factors that can both facilitate and hinder change (Burnes, 1996). The importance of considering the whole system and how its component parts interact is also emphasised (Holbeche, 2009). A systems approach is, in fact, a fundamental aspect of Human Factors and Ergonomics and this is explored in detail in the next chapter.

# References

AHRQ (2015). *Safety Program for Long-Term Care: Preventing CAUTI and Other HAIs*. Available at: www.ahrq.gov/sites/default/files/wysiwyg/professionals/quality-patient-safety/quality-resources/tools/cauti-ltc/modules/final-report.pdf.

Allcock, C. *et al.* (2015). Constructive comfort: accelerating change in the NHS. *Policy analysis, February 2015*. London: The Health Foundation.

Allegranzi, B. *et al.* (2013). 'Global implementation of WHO's multimodal strategy for improvement of hand hygiene: a quasi-experimental study' in *Lancet Infectious Diseases*, 13(10): pp. 843–851.

Barrow, J.M., Annamaraju, P., Toney-Butler, T.J. (2022). 'Change Management' in *StatPearls*. PMID: 29083813.

Berenholtz, S.M. *et al.* (2014). 'On the CUSP: Stop BSI program. Eliminating central line-associated bloodstream infections: a national patient safety imperative' in *Infection Control & Hospital Epidemiology*, 35(1): pp. 56–62.

Burden, M. (2016). 'Using a change model to reduce the risk of surgical site infection' in *British Journal of Nursing*, 25(17): pp. 949–955.

Burnes, B. (1996). 'No such thing as ... a "one best way" to manage organizational change' in *Management Decision*, 34(10): pp. 11–18.

Coghlan, A.T., Preskill, H. and Tzavaras Catsambas, T. (2003). 'An overview of appreciative inquiry in evaluation' in *New Directions for Evaluation*, 100: pp. 5–22.

Davies, H., Powell, A. and Rushmer, R. (2007). *Healthcare professionals' views on clinician engagement in quality improvement*. London: The Health Foundation.

Day, A., Crown, S.N. and Ivany, M. (2017). 'Organisational Change and Employee Burnout: The Moderating Effects of Support and Job Control' in *Safety Science*, 100: pp. 4–12.

Dixon-Woods, M. *et al.* (2011). 'Explaining Michigan: Developing an Ex-Post Theory of a Quality Improvement Program' in *Milbank Quarterly*, 89(2): pp. 167–205.

Dixon-Woods, M., McNicol, S. and Martin, G. (2012). *Overcoming challenges to improving quality*. London: The Health Foundation. Available at: www.health.org.uk/publications/overcoming-challenges-to-improving-quality/.

Dougall, D., Lewis, M. and Ross, S. (2018). *Transformational change in health and care: reports from the field*. London: The King's Fund.

Gu, Y. *et al.* (2021). 'Application of comprehensive unit-based safety program model in the inter-hospital transfer of patients with critical diseases: a retrospective controlled study' in *BMC Health Services Research*, 21(1): p. 690.

Ham, C., Berwick, D. and Dixon, J. (2016). *Improving quality in the English NHS: A strategy for action*. London: The King's Fund.

Holbeche, L. (2009). 'Organisational development — what's in a name?' in *Impact*, 26: pp. 6–9.

Hollnagel, E., Wears, R.L. and Braithwaite, J. (2015). *From Safety-I to Safety-II: A White Paper*. Available at: https://www.england.nhs.uk/signuptosafety/wp-content/uploads/sites/16/2015/10/safety-1-safety-2-whte-papr.pdf.

Hughes, R.G. (ed.) (2008). *Patient Safety and Quality: An Evidence-Based Handbook for Nurses. Agency for Healthcare Research and Quality*. Rockville (MD): Agency for Healthcare Research and Quality.

Hughes, H. (2023). 'Patient Safety, Governance, Leadership and Infection Prevention and Control' in Elliott, P., Storr, J., Jeanes, A. *Infection Prevention and Control: A Social Science Perspective*. Boda Raton: CRC Press.

IOM (2011). *The learning health system and its innovation collaboratives: Update report*. Washington, DC: The National Academies Press.

Johns Hopkins Medicine (2015). *The Comprehensive Unit-based Safety Program* (CUSP). Available at: https://www.hopkinsmedicine.org/armstrong-institute/training-services/cusp-implementation-training/cusp-guidance.

Karimi, E., Sohrabi, Z. and Aalaa, M. (2022). 'Change Management in Medical Contexts, especially in Medical Education: A Systematized Review' in *Journal of Advances in Medical Education and Professionalism*, 10(4): pp. 219–227. Doi: 10.30476/JAMP.2022.96519.1704.

Kennedy, I. (2001). *The report of the public inquiry into children's heart surgery at the Bristol Royal Infirmary 1984–1995*. Learning from Bristol (Cm 5207 (II)). HMSO; 2001. https://webarchive.national archives.gov.uk/ukgwa/20100407202128/http://www.dh.gov.uk/en/Publicationsandstatistics/Publications/PublicationsPolicyAndGuidance/DH_4005620.

Kohn, L.T., Corrigan, J.M. and Donaldson, M.S. (eds.) (1999). *To Err is Human: Building a Safer Health System*. Institute of Medicine. Washington, DC: National Academy Press.

Kotter, J.P. (2007). 'Leading Change: Why transformation efforts fail' in *Harvard Business Review*, 1: pp. 2–9.

Lipitz-Snyderman, A. *et al.* (2011). 'Impact of a statewide intensive care unit quality improvement initiative on hospital mortality and length of stay: Retrospective comparative analysis' in *British Medical Journal*, 342: d219.

Merriel, A. *et al.* (2022). 'Systematic review and narrative synthesis of the impact of Appreciative Inquiry in healthcare' in *BMJ Open Quality*, 11(2): e001911. Doi: 10.1136/bmjoq-2022-001911. PMID: 35710130; PMCID: PMC9204436.

Miller, D. (2001). 'Successful change leaders: What makes them? What do they do that is different?' in *Journal of Change Management*, 2(4): pp. 359–368.

National Academies of Sciences, Engineering, and Medicine; Health and Medicine Division; Board on Health Care Services; Board on Global Health; Committee on Improving the Quality of Health Care Globally (2018). *Crossing the Global Quality Chasm: Improving Health Care Worldwide*. Washington, DC: National Academies Press.

Noble, D.J., Lemer, C. and Stanton, E. (2011). 'What has change management in industry got to do with improving patient safety?' in *Postgraduate Medical Journal*, 87: pp. 345–348.

Patient Safety Learning (2019). *The Patient-Safe Future: A Blueprint for Action*. https://d2z1laakrytay6.cloudfront.net/content/A-Blueprint-for-Action-240619.pdf.

Phillips, J. and Klein, J.D. (2023). 'Change Management: From Theory to Practice' in *TechTrends*, 67: pp. 189–197.

Porritt, K. *et al.* (eds.) (2020). *JBI Handbook for Evidence Implementation*. JBI. https://implementation-manual.jbi.global.

Pronovost, P.J. *et al.* (2008). 'Improving patient safety in intensive care units in Michigan' in *Journal of Critical Care*, 23(2): pp. 207–21.

Pronovost, P.J. (2011). 'Navigating adaptive challenges in quality improvement'. in *BMJ Quality & Safety*, 20(7): pp. 560–3.

Ramanujam, R., Keyser, D.J. and Sirio, C.A. (2005). 'Making a Case for Organizational Change in Patient Safety Initiatives' in Henriksen, K. *et al.* (eds.) *Advances in Patient Safety: From Research to Implementation,* (vol. 2: Concepts and Methodology). Rockville (MD): Agency for Healthcare Research and Quality. PMID: 21249818.

Ratcliffe, S. (2016). *G. K. Chesterton 1874–1936: English essayist, novelist, and poet*. Oxford Essential Quotations (4th edition), Oxford University Press. Published online: www.oxfordreference.com/

display/10.1093/acref/9780191826719.001.0001/q-oro-ed4-00002890;jsessionid=6FD630DBF3E-33716BCF8743981DE72F9.

Schwarz, G.M., Bouckenooghe, D. and Vakola, M. (2021). 'Organizational change failure: framing the process of failing' in *Human Relations*, 74(2): pp. 159–179.

Shojania, K.G. and Grimshaw, J.M. (2005). 'Evidence-based quality improvement: the state of the science' in *Health Affairs*, 24(1): pp. 138–50.

Smith, R. (1998). 'All Changed, changed utterly. British medicine will be transformed by the Bristol case' in *British Medical Journal*, 27;316(7149):1912–8.

Smoyer, W.E.P. and Embi, J., Moffatt-Bruce, S. (2016). 'Creating Local Learning Health Systems: Think Globally, Act Locally' in *Journal of the American Medical Association*, 316(23): pp. 2481–2482.

Taitz, J.M., Lee, J.H. and Sequist, T.D. (2011). 'A framework for engaging physicians in quality and safety' in *BMJ Quality & Safety*, 21: pp. 722–728.

Timmel, J. *et al.* (2010). 'Impact of the Comprehensive Unit-based Safety Program (CUSP) on safety culture in a surgical inpatient unit' in *Joint Commission Journal on Quality and Patient Safety*, 36(6): pp. 252–60.

Varkey, P. and Kollengode, A. (2011). 'A framework for healthcare quality improvement in India: the time is here and now!' in *Journal of Postgraduate Medicine*, 57(3): pp. 237–41.

Vincent, C. (2010). *Patient Safety* (2nd edition). Chichester, UK: Wiley-Blackwell.

Watkins, J.M. and Cooperrider, D.L. (2000). 'Appreciative inquiry: A transformative paradigm' in *Journal of the Organization Development Network*, 32: pp. 6–12.

Weaver, S.J. *et al.* (2013). 'Promoting a culture of safety as a patient safety strategy: a systematic review' in *Annals of Internal Medicine*, 158(5 Pt 2): pp. 369–74.

Weaver, S.J. *et al.* (2015). 'A Collaborative Learning Network Approach to Improvement: The CUSP Learning Network' in *Joint Commission Journal of Quality and Patient Safety*, 41(4): pp. 147–59.

WHO (2018a). *Delivering quality health services: a global imperative for universal health coverage*. Geneva: World Health Organization, Organisation for Economic Co-operation and Development, and The World Bank.

WHO (2018b). *Taking Action: Steps 4 & 5 in Twinning Partnerships for Improvement*. Geneva: World Health Organization; (WHO/HIS/SDS/2018.14). Licence: CC BY-NC-SA 3.0 IGO.

WHO (2018c). *Preventing surgical site infections: implementation approaches for evidence-based recommendations*. Geneva: World Health Organization.

WHO (2021). *Global patient safety action plan 2021–2030: towards eliminating avoidable harm in health care*. Geneva: World Health Organization.

# CHAPTER 3

# The Systems Engineering Initiative for Patient Safety (SEIPS)
## A Human Factors Approach to Work System Analysis

*Paul Bowie and Helen Vosper*

## Summary

Human Factors and Ergonomics (HFE) as a science and practice strongly promotes a 'systems approach' to understanding healthcare interactions and related outcomes to inform the optimisation of (re)design and improvement efforts. However, knowledge and application of these principles and methods are not well-established in healthcare. The system is also lacking accessible, practical tools for all workforce levels to implement associated concepts which would pragmatically aid everyday problem-solving and inform improvement.

In this chapter, we introduce the System Engineering Initiative for Patient Safety (SEIPS) framework. SEIPS is a well-established, highly evidenced and influential Human Factors approach for identifying, understanding and analysing interactions, processes and outcomes in complex sociotechnical care systems such as much of healthcare.

Against this background, we seek to:

- Describe and define the benefits and approach of the Human Factors discipline and profession.
- Introduce and outline the guiding principles of the Human Factors 'systems approach' through use of the SEIPS framework.
- Illustrate the multi-functional application of the SEIPS framework by any care practitioner; team; leaders; educators; incident investigators; risk, safety and improvement advisors; and others in any care or educational setting.
- Discuss the potential for embedding entry-level Human Factors in everyday healthcare practice and education through the SEIPS approach.
- Provide vignettes and a case study demonstrating how SEIPS can be practically applied to problem-solving quality and safety issues in healthcare.

## Background

In the past decade, interest in embedding HFE concepts and tools in healthcare has grown significantly amongst, for example, professional bodies, regulatory agencies and higher education institutions (NHS England, 2015; WHO, 2011). HFE approaches are embedded in the work systems of many safety-critical industries worldwide because there is a strong recognition of the importance of this scientific field to the design of safe and efficient operations to reduce organisational risks and losses and enhance the health and safety of the workforce (MOD, 2015). However, knowledge and application of related concepts and methods are not well-established in the healthcare sectors, nor well-understood despite the growing interest in the field, particularly in support of patient safety education and improvement (Russ, 2013;

Hignett, 2013). Also lacking are pragmatic, accessible HFE tools that can be used by most in healthcare practice and education to aid everyday problem-solving and improvement designs with limited need for formal training (Hignett, 2013; Bowie, 2016).

One such plausible tool is SEIPS (Carayon, 2006). Although SEIPS is widely applied by health services, researchers and HFE specialists, it has significant untapped potential to be adapted for use as a practical, multi-functional work system analysis tool (Box 3.1) by most practitioners or teams, in any healthcare setting. Such a tool should also attract strong interest from specific professional groups, such as those leading and advising in clinical risk, patient safety, quality improvement, safety investigation, workforce well-being initiatives, organisational development and healthcare education and training. This also fulfils the societal ambition of many in the HFE profession 'to give ergonomics away' (Stanton, 2003) and supports the necessary goal of building related capacity and capability in the field among many in the healthcare workforce.

In this chapter, we describe the concepts underlying the SEIPS framework. It should be recognised that this is a well-established, highly evidenced and influential HFE method for identifying, understanding and analysing interactions and emergent outcomes in complex sociotechnical care systems, such as much of healthcare (Holden, 2013; Holden, 2021). To recognise the full potential of SEIPS beyond its patient safety focus and maximise its accessibility and flexibility to the aforementioned groups as a method for embedding HFE at scale across healthcare, we also demonstrate how it can be practically and flexibly applied, in combination with basic guiding principles for systems thinking (Bowie, in press). This will address a range of important work and educational activities routinely undertaken by healthcare teams.

### BOX 3.1 Examples of How the SEIPS Framework can be Applied in Healthcare

- Data collection and analysis for incident reporting and learning systems; e.g. embedding a systems-informed contributory factors classification scheme.
- Understanding work system interactions and outcomes; e.g. how any work issues combine to influence outcomes we're trying to achieve or avoid.
- Informing care system designs and redesigns; e.g. using SEIPS to think about the design of improvement interventions.
- Adopting a Human Factors approach in the design of simulation scenarios.
- Proactive systems-informed hazard identification, risk assessment and control.
- Organisational safety investigations and learning.
- Team-based learning from safety incidents, near misses, complaints and everyday work.
- Work system interactions that impact on workforce well-being; e.g. barriers and facilitators.
- Teaching the Human Factors systems approach to novice learners; e.g. undergraduate students and postgraduate trainees.
- Informing the user-centred design of work procedures; e.g. making protocols, guidance, checklists and policies relevant, usable, safer and sustainable.
- Relaying a 'system story' to senior leaders and executives.
- Problem solving everyday work system hassles, frustrations and irritations.

## The SEIPS Framework Explained

HFE as a science and practice strongly promotes a 'systems approach' (Carayon, 2006) to understanding healthcare interactions to inform the 'joint optimisation' of related work system design and improvement (Wilson, 2014). In the absence of suitable work system analysis methods for healthcare, the original SEIPS framework was specifically developed 'to advance research in, and design for, patient safety' (Figure 3.1). The framework has been updated twice in recent years, but the focus of the development described here is on the first tool published in 2006, which is arguably less complex than the other versions to engage with.

SEIPS is grounded in HFE theory and particularly in the sub-domain of macro-ergonomics, the science concerned with designing and improving overall work systems to enhance organisational performance (e.g. system safety, efficiency, productivity) and human well-being (patient safety, health and safety, experience, satisfaction, comfort, joy). This is illustrated in Figure 3.1 through its depiction of a work system that is generic and applicable to any facility in any healthcare sector (e.g. operating theatre, community pharmacy, ambulance vehicle, mental

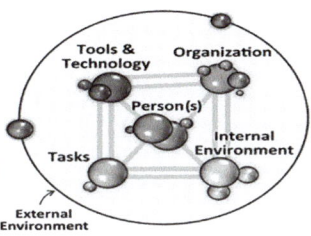

**WORK SYSTEM**

**Organisation**
- Structures external to a person (but often put in place by people) that organise time, space, resources, and activity.
- Within institutions:
  - Work schedules/staffing
  - Workload assignment
  - Management and incentive systems
  - Organisational culture (values, commitment, transparency)
  - Training
  - Policies/procedures
  - Resource availability and recruitment
- In other settings:
  - Communication infrastructure
  - Living arrangements
  - Family roles and responsibilities
  - Work and life schedules
  - Financial and health-related resources

**Tools & Technology**
Characteristics such as:
- Usability
- Accessibility
- Familiarity
- Level of automation
- Portability and functionality
- Maintenance (outdated, malfunctioning)

**Person**
- Individual characteristics:
  - Psychological impacts (e.g., frustration, stress, burnout)
  - Cognitive factors (attention, memory, confusion)
  - Preferences, personal goals
  - Knowledge, competence, skills
  - Physiological factors (illness, dehydration)
  - Physical strength and needs
- Collective characteristics: team cohesiveness

**Tasks**
- Specific actions within larger work processes
- Includes task attributes such as:
  - Difficulty
  - Complexity
  - Variety
  - Ambiguity
  - Sequence

**Internal environment**
Physical environment such as characteristics of
- Ambient environment: lighting, noise, vibration, temperature
- Physical layout and available space
- Housekeeping: cluttered, organisation, cleanliness

**External environment**
- Societal, economic, regulatory and policy factors outside an organisation

**Figure 3.1** The SEIPS Work System
Contains public sector information licensed under the Open Government Licence v3.0.

health ward, open plan offices, staff dining room). The focus of the care work system on the left of the diagram is on characterising the interactions between people and five other system elements or components: job tasks; tools and technology; the physical environment; organisation of work; and external influences such as safety legislation, regulation and policy. A fuller description of the performance influence factors related to each of these work system elements that can enhance or degrade performance and well-being is also illustrated in Figure 3.1.

It is important to note that it is the complex interactions and inter-dependencies between these system elements that combine to create both wanted and unwanted outcomes related to overall work system performance and human well-being, outlined on the right side of the diagram. The framework acknowledges that work systems and processes are dynamic and constantly adapt (illustrated by the arrows as feedback loops) and, critically, that from related work system (sometimes unpredictable) interactions, both wanted and unwanted outcomes *emerge*.

Integrated within, and aligned with all aspects of the SEIPS framework, is Donabedian's well-established conceptual model that provides a structure-process-outcomes (SPO) framework for understanding, examining, and evaluating the quality of healthcare delivery (Donabedian, 1966).

The SEIPS framework is arguably the most widely implemented, influential and evidenced HFE approach in patient safety research (Bowie, 2016). It has been flexibly applied in diverse care settings to help address a whole range of care problems; for example, to inform system-wide risk assessments; to guide development of a safety checklist; to aid analysis of identified HFE literature in primary care; and to study wrong blood in tube incidents in hospitals.

Based on the SEIPS framework, a basic worksheet with guiding notes has been developed for healthcare teams as a general problem-solving tool that can easily be adapted for use by practitioners, improvement, safety and risk advisors, researchers and educators (Figure 3.2).

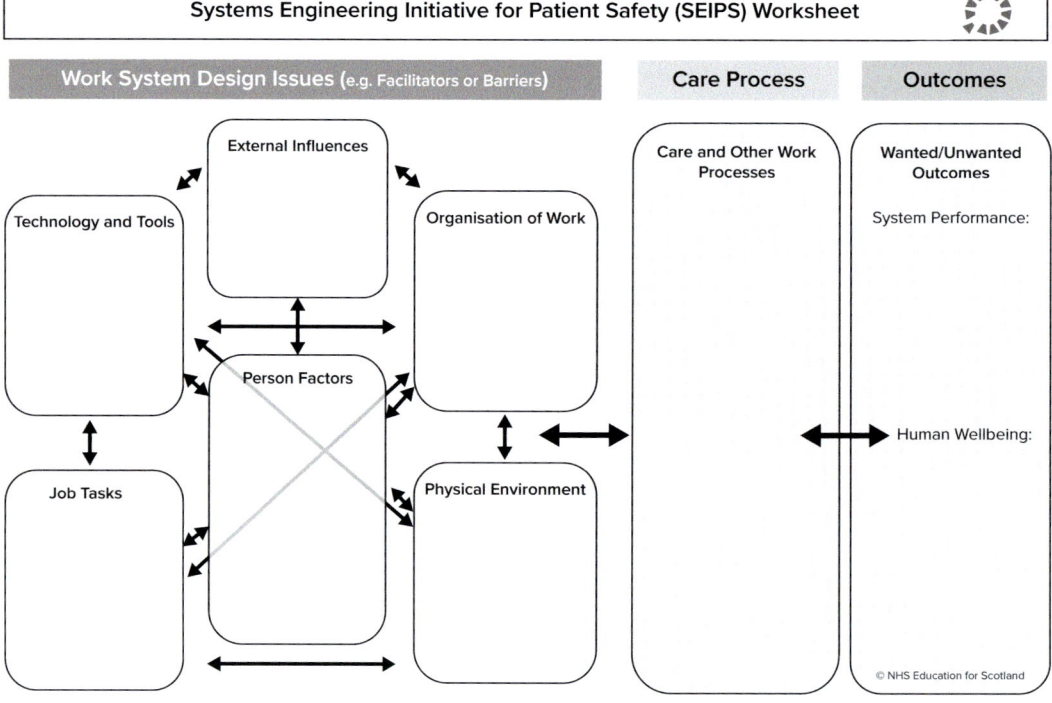

**Figure 3.2** The SEIPS Worksheet
Contains public sector information licensed under the Open Government Licence v3.0.

## Examples of the Multi-functionality of SEIPS

The following examples demonstrate where 'real-life' application of SEIPS has potential use as a systems analysis tool in diverse areas of healthcare:

### EXAMPLE 1: Data collection and analysis design for incident reporting and learning systems

Integrating systems thinking in the design and operation of incident reporting and learning systems is the predominant approach in modern safety science and in the practices of many high-risk industrial sectors but can be lacking in health and social care. The system components that comprise the SEIPS frameworks can guide the types of initial data to be collected for reportable incidents and the taxonomy of system-wide contributory factors (up to Government level) that are necessary for in-depth analysing, understanding interactions and inter-relationships and improving organisational learning.

### EXAMPLE 2: Process mapping and task analysis

SEIPS can be used on its own or in combination with other methods (e.g. hierarchical task analysis or process mapping) to provide a high-level overview of specific care processes within complex sociotechnical care systems like much of healthcare. For example, if we were to process map a local laboratory test ordering and reporting system in primary care, SEIPS can provide additional insights by identifying the higher order system components and their interactions (e.g. use of technology to enable practice-to-patient information transfer) that give rise to safe, efficient care or act as a barrier to necessary system performance.

### EXAMPLE 3: Care system redesign (pharmacy)

The application of a 'systems approach' is recommended in the design or redesign of care systems as part of improvement work and SEIPS provides a simple but powerful framework to support such an approach. Case study research aimed at improving the positive impact on the performance of pharmacists working in a general medical practice setting identified how interactions between the different aspects of SEIPS influenced their performance, for example:

- *Person* — cognitive preferences and personal goals influenced efficiency and thoroughness.
- *Tasks* — certain tasks suited a defined thorough approach, whereas others involved varying responses and dealing with high levels of uncertainty often at odds with goals set for pharmacists.
- *Technology* — access to suitable technology was variable but helped reduce uncertainty with a resultant reduction in workload for pharmacists and other sectors of healthcare.
- *Internal environment* — varying the positioning of pharmacists so they worked with multiple different team members increased their understanding of the system, altered their goal orientation and how they processed tasks to increase efficiency.
- *Organisation* — work schedules and policies (such as over specified protocols) limited the ability of pharmacists to adapt performance to optimise both efficiency and thoroughness.
- *External influences* — national policy promoted the ability of pharmacists to increase quality, reduce workload and make cost efficiency savings. These were often competing goals and trade-offs between goals depended on pharmacists' cognitive preferences, goals, assigned tasks, understanding of the system and organisational set-up.

Exploration of the interactions between these factors led to the development of system-wide recommendations to redesign systems to improve performance and well-being.

## EXAMPLE 4: Hazard identification, risk assessment and control

Taking a systems approach to risk assessment and control is recommended in all industries. SEIPS can facilitate this process by prompting healthcare teams and risk assessors to go beyond the traditional focus on people and think more holistically across the different system elements where hazards (things that may cause harm) may lurk and where consequently people may be harmed, and care organisations suffer losses. For example, when converting non-care buildings or designing bespoke facilities to support mass Covid-19 vaccination rollouts, SEIPS was applied to examine in detail the potential system-wide issues that may pose risks and that need to be managed, such as:

- At the person-level (e.g. patient mobility).
- For tools and technology (e.g. cold chain storage problems or the usability of supporting digital apps for data capture).
- The physical environments (e.g. ingress and egress of patients and others).
- External influences (e.g. pharmaceutical supply and availability of vaccines or national immunisation policies).

## EXAMPLE 5: Teaching basic Human Factors

One of the problems with current health and care understanding of HFE is the conflation between Human Factors and 'factors of the human' (Vosper, 2018). This has largely arisen from a lack of understanding of the origin of non-technical skills training in aviation. In aviation, HFE is embedded throughout, to the point at which much of this is invisible to frontline staff. A systems analysis of a number of accidents revealed that non-technical skills as person factors (to use SEIPS terminology) were major contributory factors. This led to the development of Crew Resource Management (CRM), which has been enthusiastically taken up in health and care. However, if a systems analysis has not been undertaken to identify non-technical skills as a problem for a given system, then CRM type training is not Human Factors! SEIPS is therefore useful in teaching the fundamentals of HFE to healthcare staff. It can be used to both address the conflation and to introduce the learner to essential systems thinking principles.

## EXAMPLE 6: Workforce well-being

We can apply SEIPS to identify, map and examine the different system-wide psychosocial hazards that contribute to increased work-related stress and levels of burnout among different groups of staff (e.g. hospital doctors-in-training). Systemic contributory factors associated with burnout may include issues such as complex and emotionally demanding job tasks; high levels of workload; lack of food facilities and accommodation; the use of digital technologies; the prevailing safety culture in a specific clinical unit; and the impact on frontline work of external policy targets. SEIPS can therefore be used as a proactive work system analysis tool to identify these psychosocial hazards, assess risks and put in place control measures.

## SEIPS and Basic Systems Thinking Principles

In addition to the adaptation of key SEIPS framework content, the following systems thinking principles further guide users when applying the tool:

1. Define your local system 'boundary' to make it more manageable (you cannot solve everything).
2. Seek out the experiences and views of others regardless of seniority or work role as they have different perspectives on how the system works and can be improved.
3. Recognise that care delivery will result in both wanted and unwanted outcomes because of the highly complex, multiple, interacting contributory factors from across the system, not just the decisions and actions of a single person.

4. When looking back at the decisions and actions of others involved in, for example, safety incidents or the design of care systems, do not blame or judge but seek to understand why these made sense given both the context and situation they faced at the time, otherwise they would not have made them (this is known as the local rationality principle).
5. Explore the differences and seek to close the gap between work as imagined — i.e. what is written in policies and guidance and assumed in the minds of those removed from the 'sharp-end'; and work as done — i.e. how that work is done in reality at the 'coalface' of everyday healthcare practice.
6. Finally, focus learning and improvement on wider systemic design solutions as much as possible and less so on person-level behavioural interventions or weak or passive recommendations or improvement interventions. (For example, asking people to remember to do things to improve the reliability of a care process is unlikely to be sustained, nor is introducing an improvement that will add a few minutes work to their day.)

## Comparison Between SEIPS and the Fishbone Diagram (Figure 3.3)

When first introduced to SEIPS, many improvement advisors and others often compare and erroneously conflate the approach with the Fishbone diagram. From a QI perspective, there is the potential for confusion and misunderstanding regarding the relationship between the SEIPS framework and 'similar' system analysis tools, such as the Fishbone diagram — a technique widely taught and applied in QI (including safety investigations). Although both approaches may appear at first sight to take a comparable 'systems approach' there are marked differences in the underlying system assumptions and perspectives for each tool and it is vitally important to highlight these.

For SEIPS, a clear focus is on identifying the complex *interactions* and *inter-relationships* between work system components and how these function as barriers to, or facilitators of, both wanted and unwanted outcomes related to system performance and human well-being. (The joint optimisation of these important outcomes aligns perfectly with the 'twin aims' of Human Factors science and practice.) In the SEIPS perspective, healthcare systems interactions are highly complex, often unpredictable, and related outcomes are viewed as *emergent* phenomena that result from these, sometimes unpredictable and unforeseeable, interactions. (For example, 'patient safety' does not reside in a single system component, such as a clinician or a checklist, but emerges from the interactions of multiple, system elements.)

In contrast, the philosophy and assumptions underlying the Fishbone diagram (Ishikawa, 1990) are different. The work system is arguably viewed in reductionist terms as being simple, tractable, static and predictable, and each component can largely be identified and understood in terms of how it relates to other components and then 'fixed'. There is a lack of focus on guiding the user to study complex interactions and a key goal is to identify a single outcome (e.g. a 'root cause') that is assumed to be the result of linear 'cause and effect' relationships. Overall, the approach attempts to understand highly complex issues in simplistic terms, without guiding the user to consider complexity, interactions and inter-dependencies, feedback loops, emergence and the outcome focus being on BOTH performance and well-being.

| System Assumptions of SEIPS | System Assumptions of Fishbone Diagram |
| --- | --- |
| • Complex, intractable and adaptive | • Simple, tractable and static |
| • Unpredictable | • Predictable |
| • Dynamic, non-linear interactions | • Linear cause and effect |
| • Multiple, interlinked outcomes | • 'Root cause' / single effect |
| • Emergence | • Reductionist |

**Figure 3.3** System Assumptions of SEIPS and the Fishbone Diagram

## Application of SEIPS: the NHS Health Check

The application of SEIPS was used as part of the NHS Health Check. The NHS Health Check is an English service in which all those over the age of 40 years are invited for an assessment of their individual 10-year cardiovascular risk. This has made it useful for studying when taking a Human Factors approach. A detailed client history is taken and some simple tests are carried out, including blood pressure, body mass index and blood lipid measurements. These data are entered into a risk engine and the resultant 10-year risk is used to inform the development of a plan to reduce cardiovascular risk.

This example refers to the Health Check in the community pharmacy setting. The Health Check is one part of the national cardiovascular risk management strategy that can be considered as the macro system, whereas the Health Check itself is a meso-level system nesting within that macro-system. A Human Factors approach was taken to exploring the Health Check. Data came from direct observation (and Hierarchical Task Analysis (HTA)), but also from interviews and focus groups with staff and clients. This data suggested that many of the problems that might undermine the success of the Health Check actually occur at the macro-level; it was clear that staff struggled to carry out all the activities in the time that was allocated.

When this was discussed in focus groups and interviews, it turned out that the payment the pharmacy receives for these additional services is quite small and, if the time could not be controlled, it was possible that money would be lost. Current national policy and strategy is actively encouraging pharmacists to take on more clinical roles. However, the remuneration model seems to largely reward dispensing. Probably the most effective recommendation would be to change this — if you want pharmacists to offer additional clinical services, we would need to pay them for it. However, change will take time and so the need to focus on what could be controlled was recognised.

The Health Check is task heavy and so the best strategy would be to consider how performance in each of the individual tasks can be improved. Each task can be considered a micro-system, nesting within the meso-system. The SEIPS analysis shown here is for the task of blood lipid measurement. Data showed it to be problematic in multiple ways. In fact, it was common for this task not to be completed. Given the importance of the total:high density lipoprotein (HDL) cholesterol ratio in predicting cardiovascular risk, this wasn't good. Focusing on this one task allowed boundaries to be set.

Some of the system entities relating to lipid measurement are shown in Figure 3.4. 'People' included the pharmacist and the client. The 'task' of measuring the blood lipids can be broken down into several subtasks. We could go into much more detail here, but it has been limited to just a few steps for clarity — these are things the SEIPS analysis has identified as important. Your first SEIPS analysis is likely to identify many entities, some of which are likely to be removed later when you decide they are not relevant. Do not worry about this — accept it will be an iterative process. Similarly, we have only listed the equipment that we believe influences the outcomes in some way.

Let us look at what we mean by interactions. We have already identified that the need to be profitable limits the amount of time available for tasks. This is our first interaction (a task–organisation interaction). Based on this important interaction, we can see that to get a successful result, we need to streamline the task as much as possible. This does not mean 'just try to work faster' — that is unlikely to be successful. However, by deconstructing it, we can see if we can redesign the task to make it faster.

The data from HTA suggested multiple possibilities. The biggest by far was that many of the pharmacies were using machines that only measure one lipid at a time, requiring a separate blood sample for each. The readings also took a couple of minutes each, eating into the total time available. This is a task-technology interaction: the design of the technology means that we need an extra step in the task. We could improve this interaction by using a different piece of equipment — one which can measure both total and HDL cholesterol from the same blood sample. You might not be able to do anything about this immediately, but you can file the information for the next time there is a procurement opportunity.

Often, interactions occur between more than two entities at the same time. If we consider the task–tool interaction we have just highlighted, it could be complicated by a further interaction with the client. We observed that people could be quite squeamish about having a blood sample taken. They might just about manage the first one, but on several occasions, they refused the second one! In this case, it would be a person–technology–task interaction.

| Pharmacist  Client | Take blood sample  Apply to stick  Read  REPEAT | Lancet etc  Disposable pipette  Reflotron  Computer | Procurement process  Need to be profitable | Ambient temperature |
|---|---|---|---|---|

**Figure 3.4** System Entities for Blood Lipid Measurement

Another important interaction is related to the design of the disposable pipette used to collect the specific volume of blood that needs to be applied to the test stick. These pipettes are poor, and the blood refused to be drawn up into the pipette and just clotted. This task–tool interaction could be overcome by using a proper pipette. There are other interactions we could consider, even based on this simplified table. For example, we often observed that warm environments meant that blood flowed easily for sampling (an example of a good person–environment–task interaction) and that a reassuring, personable pharmacist could overcome client anxiety (a person–person interaction).

How did we know which interactions were the most important and therefore the ones we could choose to discuss? This is exactly the same as for any other data analysis. Frequency is important (so the interactions mentioned are ones we saw happening repeatedly). But it's also important to consider the potential to cause harm. Given that the total:HDL ratio is one of the most important indicators of risk available (something we know from the literature and from the NICE Guidelines that underpin the Health Check), not taking this reading could result in missing a client who is at high risk of a cardiovascular event.

## Final Thoughts

SEIPS is strongly recommended as a highly evidence-based conceptual framework and method for taking a Human Factors-based approach to patient safety research and evaluation. However, as hopefully illustrated, it has arguably even greater potential as an accessible and flexible HFE tool for those at the 'sharp end' of healthcare as well as educators teaching entry-level HFE with the addition of fundamental systems thinking principles to guide its implementation in context. If widely adopted, there is strong potential for embedding entry-level HFE in everyday care practice and education through this approach and helping to spread this type of flexible, multi-functional approach to applying the 'systems approach' to problem-solving and organisational learning.

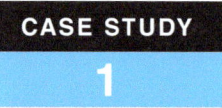 **CASE STUDY 1** — Vicky Baker, Patient Safety Lead for a Healthcare Provider that Delivers Community and Offender Healthcare Services on Behalf of the NHS and Local Authority Public Health Services.

## Background

The patient safety lead had completed a thematic review of root cause analysis (RCA) investigations and noted several repeat recommendations around care planning.

Although the completed RCA investigation was comprehensive, the recommendations were not aligned to a systems approach to investigations; recommendations were often focused on individual staff making changes. Examples of recurrent recommendations related to care planning were:

'Staff must ensure that patients have completed care plans.'
'Staff must ensure that care plans are completed in a timely manner.'
'Staff must ensure that care plans are individualised.'

As a learning organisation, we wanted to understand why recommendations that had been completed were not having an impact on practice and why they were resulting in repeat recommendations being made.

To improve this, we decided to use a systems approach to understand the contributing factors related to sub-optimal care planning management. The SEIPS model was used as it is a system approach specifically designed for use within complex healthcare settings. Additionally, the organisation had taken the steps to actively promote this model as a way of investigating incidents so there was emerging familiarity with some staff across the organisation.

## What We Did

Initially, the patient safety lead shared findings of the thematic reviews through our internal local governance groups and subcommittees to the board. We already had buy-in from our senior management and executive team to use a systems thinking approach to investigations as this was an agreed objective within our patient safety strategy.

The patient safety lead set up a workshop, promoted through the internal communication department and attendance at various internal governance meetings, with a view that clinical staff would attend to discuss the barriers to care planning and provide that vital work as done narrative to everyday care planning.

Prior to the meeting, a planning event was held between the patient safety lead and a Human Factors specialist commissioned to work with the organisation over a 12 month period to promote the use of systems thinking within the organisation. We agreed to use a SEIPS model but adapted the framework slightly. Within the SEIPS model, the outcomes box is usually used to capture the outcome of a process, considering the work system areas identified (see Figure 3.5). For this workshop, we used the outcomes box to determine with the group what 'good care planning would look like' for the organisation, the patient and staff.

At the workshop an initial introduction was given to outline that the purpose of the workshop was to understand from a systems perspective the barriers impacting on care planning. An overview of SEIPS was provided explaining the different areas. We explained to the group that initially we would be capturing 'what good looks like' by completing the outcomes section.

The first stage of the workshop worked well, with lots of staff engagement helping to articulate the standards expected. It also helped capture staff and patient well-being when care planning is working well.

The workshop went on to capture the barriers to care planning. This was captured by the completion of the systems area of SEIPS (the 'Work System' section in Figure 3.5). In the spirit of a just culture, staff were encouraged to share their experiences at the workshop with a view that this was a learning experience to improve practice from a systems perspective rather than focusing on individual practice. See Figure 3.5 for the completed SEIPS.

We also shared with the workshop the examples of SEIPS work system descriptors so staff less familiar with SEIPS could gain an understanding of different factors in each area (see Figure 3.6).

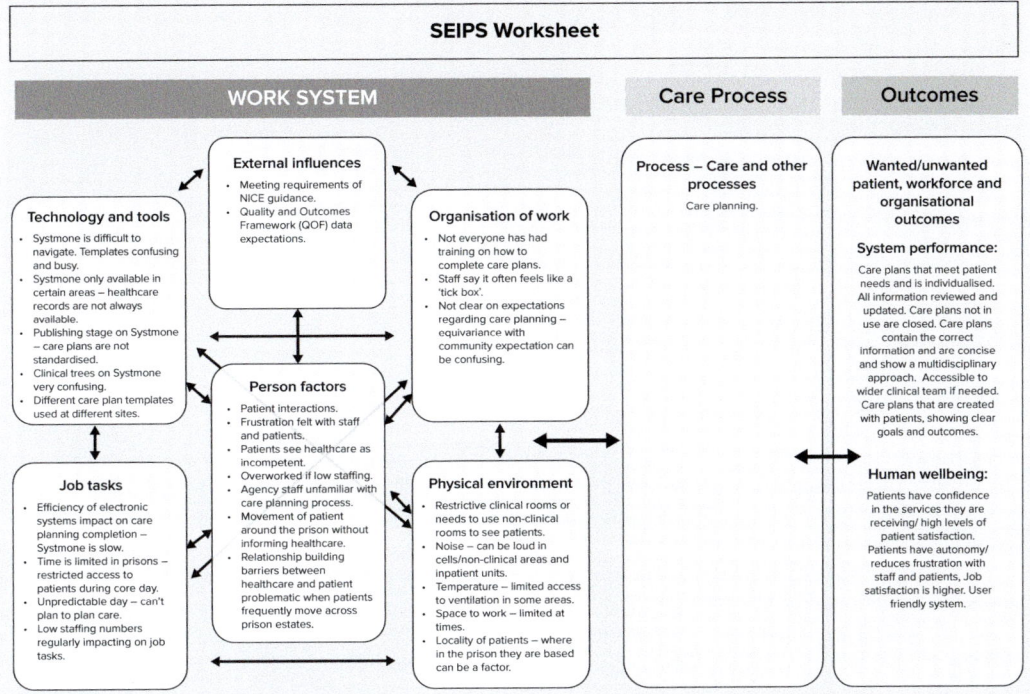

Figure 3.5 Completed SEIPS Model

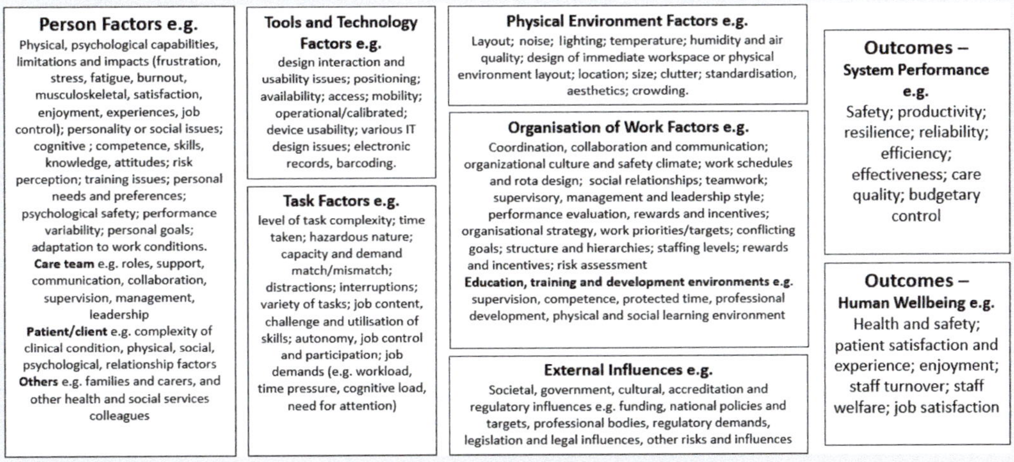

Figure 3.6 SEIPS Example of Work System Descriptors

The structure of the SEIPS model was displayed on screen while a facilitated discussion was supported by going through each area. The person factors were left until last so that everyone could see the populated areas that might impact on a person. This stage of the workshop was slow to start, with staff needing prompting to consider examples that could be relevant in each area; however, as the conversations started, this generated others to join in.

## Lessons Learned

The workshop went well, staff engaged in the process and were keen to share their experiences and highlight barriers to care planning. This created an opportunity for staff engagement and an opportunity for clinical staff to share their frustrations and suggestions of how things could be improved.

The use of the outcomes section in SEIPS to help determine 'what good looked like' was a useful introduction to the workshop. In this case, we were reviewing care planning from a general perspective rather than from a specific incident; we already knew the patient outcomes from the thematic review that had previously been completed.

## Evaluation and Impact

The outcome of the completed SEIPS workshop identified several systems contributing factors:

- IT equipment availability
- limitations of the working environment
- usability of the clinical systems
- staff training as key systemic issues.

IT equipment availability and work environments were less controllable actions as these related to the settings in which clinical staff work; for example, the work environment is limited to set clinical hours and IT equipment are in fixed areas of the organisation. The IT department is seeking solutions related to the possible use of mobile tablet devices.

Following the SEIPS workshop, the section of the action plan shown in Figure 3.7 highlights the systems actions relating to care planning work streams. The SEIPS template supports the identification of factors contributing to care plan delivery from a wider systems perspective. However, an analysis of the completed SEIPS tool was required to make system recommendations. The SEIPS template illustrated in Figure 3.5 does not provide a section to capture next steps/action plans; therefore, this was captured on a separate SMART (Specific, Measurable, Achievable, Realistic and Timely) plan (see Figure 3.7).

| Recommendation | Action Required in SMART Format | Responsible Lead (Their initials & role) |
| --- | --- | --- |
| Review of Systmone care plans to support a user-friendly interface. | 1. Standardisation of care plans for the organisation to use.<br>2. Robust governance processes to support care plan template management.<br>3. Template usability testing to take place with clinical staff to promote ease of use. | Head of performance |
| Ensure training for Systmone is available to all staff via various means. | 1. Care plan training in place at induction of new staff.<br>2. Care plan training packages available to all staff via intranet page.<br>3. Systmone champions in all sites. | Head of performance |

**Figure 3.7** Snapshot of SMART Action Plan

## Conclusions

This was the first time we had completed a workshop using a systems approach. Although our organisation has been promoting the use of SEIPS theory, using it in practice required someone that was familiar with SEIPS to be able to facilitate the session.

The use of prompt questions for each section was used as an introduction and everyone had a copy of the SEIPS prompt work sheet. Going forward, we are using SEIPS more regularly and staff familiarity and confidence in its use is growing.

The action plan (Figure 3.7) saw a shift from recommendations being team-focused or staff-focused, which had little impact, to a wider piece of work focusing on improving the interface and usability of the care plan templates. This work captured both a systems perspective and the Human Factors element of an IT user interface.

---

**CASE STUDY 2** — Victoria Wills, Head of Human Factors and Patient Safety Systems, Safety Department, Gloucestershire Hospitals NHS Foundation Trust

## Background

In April 2021, Gloucestershire Hospitals NHS Foundation Trust (GHNHSFT) reported two patient safety incidents that met the criteria for a 'never event'. This took the number of never events within Trauma and Orthopaedics to six since March 2019. Never events are defined as

> 'Serious Incidents that are wholly preventable because guidance or safety recommendations that provide strong systematic barriers are available' (NHS Improvement, 2018).

Such events require a patient safety investigation to be undertaken to identify the contributory factors and make recommendations for improvements to prevent the event from reoccurring (NHS England, 2015). This was the approach that had been taken by GHNHSFT; however, the improvement was not being achieved and as such, similar events were reported.

With PSIRF laying the foundations for system-based analysis and improvement, it presented an opportunity for an alternative approach, changing from a focus on the undesired outcomes to the system from which they were produced.

The approach we used was the SEIPS (Carayon *et al.*, 2006) and CARe QI (Anderson and Ross, 2020) to explore the system and identify opportunities to build system resilience. Staff were supported in applying a QI approach (Langley *et al.*, 2009) to the findings from the systems analysis to develop and test interventions based on the reality of 'work as done' (Hollnagel *et al.*, 2015).

## What We Did

### System Analysis

With the scope of the review defined as 'procedures within trauma and orthopaedic theatres, which use implants', staff were supported to create process maps that described the current process, starting with the identification of a suitable patient through to their post operative recovery. These were created virtually, due to restrictions in place during the Covid-19 pandemic, before being recreated using Microsoft Word and provided to the theatre staff for review. Due to the variation and complexity in theatre processes, the process maps were recognised to represent 'work as imagined', however, they provided a sufficiently representative outline of the processes, such that the scope of the system under review could be confirmed and the analysis could be planned.

A workshop was held for approximately 40 multidisciplinary staff from theatres. The staff were separated into seven groups, representing different parts of the process, which had been identified by the process maps. Allocation was decided based on subject matter expertise, whilst trying to ensure that each group had representation from each professional group. The participants were introduced to SEIPS and then, facilitated by members of the Trust patient safety team, asked to identify the elements of the system under review, describe how theses elements interacted and their resulting outcomes.

Once the SEIPS framework had been used to review the system, observational studies of the same system were planned using CARe QI. The aim was to move away from documenting 'work as imagined' and instead to try and discover 'work as done', with a particular focus on understanding the resilience of the system being studied. Staff who were willing to act as observers were identified and took part in a virtual briefing on the CARe QI handbook, covering how to conduct and document the observations. Observations were planned across the seven elements of the trauma and orthopaedic processes that had been identified through process mapping and reviewed using SEIPS. Observations were recorded on the worksheets provided by the CARe QI handbook and, where necessary, staff were asked questions to understand further what was being observed.

The theatre team morning brief was used to communicate to staff that an observational study was under way and to reassure staff that its aim was to identify opportunities for improvement, not to assess individual performance.

Once completed, the worksheets were returned and reviewed with the aim of identifying any evidence of the resilience indicators (anticipation, learning, adaptation, monitoring, responding and coordinating) highlighted by CARe QI, within the system under review. Additionally, information on system outcomes and indications of misalignments in demand and capacity were noted. These resilience indicators were then used to construct a resilience narrative, which was used to identify opportunities for improvement of further analysis.

## *Quality Improvement*

The transition from system analysis into system improvement, was supported through a QI collaborative, run by the Gloucestershire Safety and Quality Improvement Academy (GSQIA). As part of this collaborative, twenty multidisciplinary theatre staff embarked on five QI projects, focused on building system resilience in the areas identified through the analysis.

The collaborative was initiated by a day of QI training based on the Model for Improvement (Langley et al., 2009), delivered virtually. Each project developed an aim, change ideas that were tested using PDSA cycles and a measurement strategy that enabled the team to identify whether the change resulted in actual improvement. Figure 3.8 depicts the tools that were used.

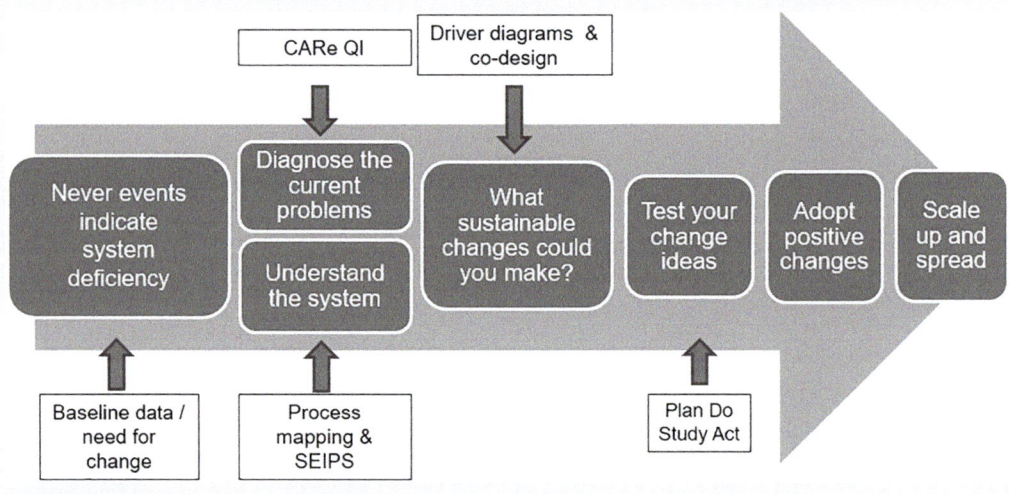

**Figure 3.8** Linking System Analysis with Quality Improvement

Teams were allocated a QI coach and Human Factors support, to work with them over the nine months that their projects spanned. The collaborative concluded in September 2022, with the teams presenting their projects at a sharing and celebration event.

Whilst the collaborative supported the findings from the system review that required an improvement approach, other areas highlighted by the study required management review or action, whilst some required audit to validate if change was required. Whilst the QI projects were progressed and supported through the QI collaborative these other actions were progressed and monitored through the never event governance meeting.

## Lessons Learned

Diverse views related to the system that the staff were working in were able to be collected through the use of SEIPS, while the observational approach of the CARe QI handbook enabled the adaptations and variations that were occurring within the system to be witnessed, such that the system diagnosis could capture the gap between 'work as imagined' and 'work as done'. These approaches in combination helped to describe the complexity of the system and the reality of work as done, while recognising the value of engaging staff in the analysis and improvement processes.

The change in approach supported a broader review, leading to the identification of contributors and associated opportunities for improvement that had not been highlighted previously by the traditional Safety-I investigation processes undertaken by GHNHSFT. This supports the findings from those such as Anderson and Watt (2020), Hollnagel *et al.* (2015) and Wiig *et al.* (2020) who have highlighted the limitations of the investigation process.

## Limitations

This system review was undertaken during the COVID-19 pandemic and as such was impacted by restrictions on group gatherings and staff availability, due to sickness. As such, the following modification were made:

- The teams taking part in the SEIPS workshop were distributed across different rooms to limit the number and proximity of people within one space. This may have impacted the opportunity for knowledge sharing and interaction.
- The core component of QI teaching was delivered virtually over Microsoft Teams, instead of a face-to-face workshop.

Staff shortages contributed to an increase in the anticipated time that the system review and its associated improvement took. It also impacted on the number of observations undertaken, potentially limiting the opportunities to view 'work as done'. This issue was replicated in the progress of the improvement projects, as participation was impacted by the ongoing need to staff theatre lists.

The use of CARe QI enabled 'work as done' to be observed, however it was not possible for this to represent all shifts, days of the week, teams at work or variation in process. Therefore, the observations only represented a sample of the system at work and so may not have been representative of all permutations or captured all factors that limited system resilience.

Similarly, any issues that were observed may have been overrepresented due to the limited sample size of the observations conducted. This risk was mitigated to some extent by using two system analysis tools so that their outputs could be compared. No anomalies were identified by this comparison.

To enable this approach to be applied in practice, the system under review was split into sections. This prevented an entirely holistic approach, but was a necessary adaptation to enable the tools to be applied in practice across a complex system. Whilst the Trust safety department coordinated this work, this was done in collaboration with a member of the theatre team, who brought departmental knowledge which was essential to the planning and implementation of the approach.

This approach required a compromise between breadth of study and the time available. The development, agreement and implementation of this approach took significantly longer than a standard 60-day serious incident investigation.

Due to the SI framework still being in place when this review was undertaken, an investigation report was produced within the required 60-day timescale, however the recommendations included in the report, referred to the outputs and improvement projects from the system safety review. Having the time and permission to enact this approach without the development of the standard action plan was agreed with the Trust executive team, the clinical commissioning group (CCG) and the care quality commission (CQC).

## Evaluation and Impact

Through the process maps, four stages of the elective orthopaedic and three stages of the trauma process were identified, these are described in Table 3.1.

**Table 3.1** Scope of System Review

| Elective Orthopaedic | Trauma |
|---|---|
| 1. Patient and implant identification, pre-assessment and listing. | 1. Day before and day of procedure: Trauma list creation and amendment process. |
| 2. Implant request, stock check and preparation. | 2. Day of procedure: Pre-list and pre-procedure implant checks. |
| 3. Day of procedure: Implant collection and checking prior to patient arrival. | 3. During procedure: In-theatre implant checks. |
| 4. Day of procedure: Implant checks prior to fit for trays/sterile packaged components and loan items. | |

The process stages were used to describe the scope of the SEIPS analysis and the observations. Each stage was allocated to an observer, with some observers covering more than one stage.

The resilience narratives constructed from the observations were compared with the SEIPS analysis before being used to formulate the following recommendations identified in Table 3.2.

**Table 3.2** Actions Recommended by CARe QI

| | |
|---|---|
| QI Project | Increase the successful completion of pre-assessment activities for elective orthopaedic cases. |
| | Improve the timely communication of necessary list changes within the two-week list 'lockdown' for elective trauma and orthopaedic cases. |
| | Improving the storage of implants within theatres and the alignment of stock held with usage requirements. |
| | Improve the in-theatre checking process for implants. |
| | Improve the resilience of the 'golden patient' identification and notification, as part of the trauma list creation process. |
| Management Review | Review the demands on the role of the theatre coordinator. |
| | Review the impact of theatre utilisation requirements. |
| | Review capacity and demand of X-ray provision in theatres. |
| | Risk review of staffing and skill mix accounting for case demand and complexity. |
| Audit | Assess the availability and provision of sets for expected case load. |
| | Assess the consistency of staff inclusion in the pre-list WHO briefing. |

As this approach was triggered by never events within trauma and orthopaedic theatres, their reoccurrence and frequency were monitored as part of this overall review. Following this period of work and at the time of writing (February 2023) it has been 422 days since the last never event in theatres. Although this represents a significant increase in time between never events, it is not possible to attribute this to the system safety review alone, due to the lack of a control group for comparison and the many variables within the operational environment of theatres.

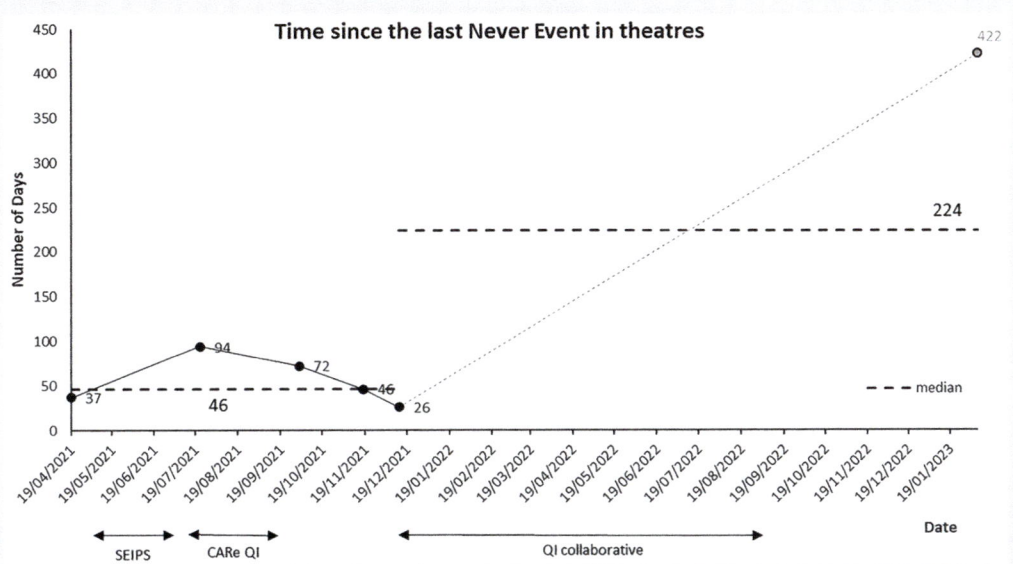

**Figure 3.9** Time Since Last Never Event in Theatres

## Conclusions

The system safety review required time, staff engagement, planning and coordination to change the focus from describing work as imagined to discovering work as done. This type of approach is supported by the introduction of PSIRF but will require a change in organisational expectations and outputs. The application of this approach demonstrated the many benefits of systems approaches including their ability to highlight the adaptability of staff, the complexity of systems and the discrepancy that exists between work as imagined and work as done. These approaches also demonstrate the value of staff involvement and engagement in improvement efforts and that the combined application of approaches such as, SEIPS, CARe QI and QI methodology, can be used to develop the proportionate system-based approaches introduced by PSIRP.

## CASE STUDY 3

Anonymous, NHS Secondary Care Provider

### Background

Given the advent of PSIRF, my Trust needed to decide on its approach to patient safety incident investigations (PSII). There were many different approaches discussed and, although we are still deliberating the best way forward, this example shows how we conducted a PSII coordinated from a central patient safety and improvement team.

Data had suggested that there may have been an issue in our laboratory sample pathway — between the sample being taken from the patient and it reaching the laboratory — as a number of samples had gone missing. Because of the large number of interacting elements and the complexity of the laboratory pathway, we decided to use this to pilot the new PSII methodology using our new SEIPS-themed process map and observations template. We felt that the other alternative learning responses and tools would not have been sufficient to capture all the interactions and influencing factors on this pathway.

By completing this pilot, we wanted to:

- Prove our new methodology worked and make any required changes. This would allow us to finalise the process and optimise the outcomes before sharing this more widely; both internally and externally.
- Explore the practicalities of SEIPS/systems thinking to discover influencing factors on the pathways and highlight various elements for the next stage of the PSII: data, people to interview and documentation used across the pathway.

### What We Did

Initially, we used the NHS England PSII template to highlight what we would need to collect to be able to complete the report template and this was then written into a flowchart. Conducting this PSII as an external team to the process meant that we did not have the same understanding of the process as those involved in the service. This impacted our ability to identify data sources, people for interviews, processes to observe and any relevant documentation.

We added a SEIPS-themed process map step into the flowchart (Figure 3.10). A traditional process map uses different coloured sticky notes to note down steps in a process, identify problems, systems/tools etc. and once it is in the correct order can be converted to an electronic format. This is a process that the team were very familiar with conducting and thus making some minor modifications to make the process SEIPS-focused was not likely to cause any issue.

A new standard operating procedure (SOP) was written for conducting a SEIPS-focused process map that would allow influencing factors to be identified. The following SEIPS elements were captured:

- Steps in the process (tasks): yellow sticky notes.
- Any issues identified at each step: pink sticky notes under the corresponding yellow.
- People: identified on the yellow notes along with task.
- Technology and tools (including documentation), physical environment, organisation: coloured dot on the corresponding sticky note.
- Ideas for improvement: blue sticky notes.

The full patient safety team was involved in the creation and running of the new style process map, which created ownership over the process rather than having to get people to buy into the process. We made sure that senior staff were updated regularly by reporting progress at the regular safety meeting that senior staff from across the organisation attended.

After the process map was completed, observations of various parts of the process were conducted. The purpose of this was to gain an understanding from an external perspective as to where issues may lie. We conducted the observations using parts of the NHS England Learning Response tool kit in conjunction with an internal document and a SEIPS template also prepared by NHSE. This is illustrated in Figure 3.2.

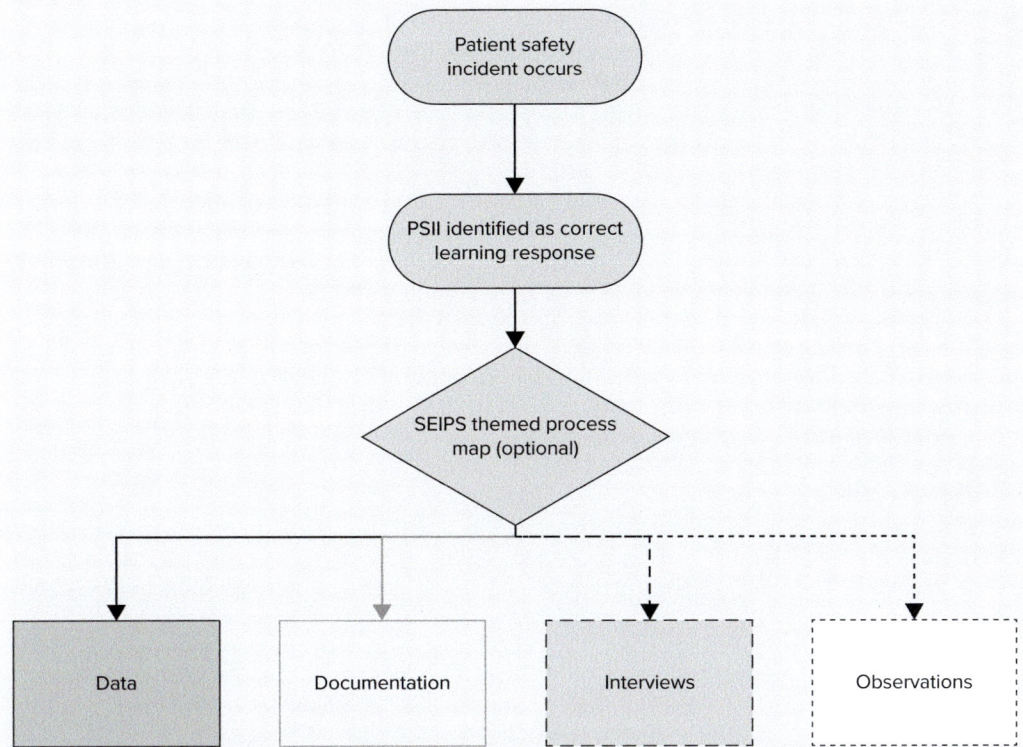

**Figure 3.10** SEIPS-Themed Process Maps Added to a Flowchart

## Lessons Learned

One of the biggest challenges we faced was getting staff involved in the process to take ownership of it. As a safety team, we spent a lot of time chasing and organising the PSII process and ensuring that the correct people were available to represent the various areas in the process. As we will need to carry out more PSIIs and we only have a small patient safety and improvement team, we will need to create increased ownership from teams and departments over involvement of the PSII process with support from the safety team rather than the process being driven by them. The alternative would be to completely change our model and look at funding a central investigation team, which has not been discussed at this point. This is a challenge that is likely to be faced across organisations due to the pressure on resources faced in the health sector.

Another challenge we encountered was the shift from looking at incidents from a root cause perspective to looking at things from a systems perspective. This challenge was in part combatted by using the SEIPS templates provided by NHS England. These helped to guide the team through the process and focus thinking on the relevant elements within the process. By using these as a template to conduct and write up our observations, we had an effective prompt to facilitate the inclusion of the various factors.

Considering processes from a SEIPS perspective was a relatively new way of working for everyone involved. Despite the challenges, the data and observations that were made were detailed and gave a holistic view of the system that the work was carried out in. The results that we managed to gather will prove invaluable to the writing of the PSII report.

## Evaluation and Impact

As a result of using the SEIPS model we were able to collect well organised, valuable information and evaluate the whole work system rather than looking at processes in isolation. The model guided us to look at factors that influence outcomes and make an evaluation of these. As a result, we have gathered a variety of evidence that will contribute to writing the PSII report.

Throughout the process, each stage was documented in an accessible way. The process map was typed and saved and the actions recorded. Observations were recorded in writing before being typed directly into a SEIPS template. This meant that the whole team had access to the documents, and we could manage the next steps and report writing.

For those involved in the pilot it supported their professional development in terms of developing knowledge of systems thinking and gaining a working knowledge of this theoretical framework. This exercise has consolidated learning since the introduction of PSIRF and facilitated the development of practical skills after undertaking an online SEIPS based training course.

These practical skills will allow us to add experience to the training that we are developing internally for staff on the systems thinking learning responses presented by PSIRF. This training will be rolled out to those that are likely to be involved in incident investigation and being able to talk from experience will add a richness to the training, helping us to embed this way of thinking across the organisation to promote a patient safety culture.

## Conclusions

The advice we would offer to anyone who is looking to complete a similar piece of work is to take advantage of the templates that have been provided online by NHS England and tailor these to suit your organisation. The templates were invaluable in guiding our thinking and documentation of the results.

We would recommend creating ownership and getting buy-in early in the process. This is a new way of working and there is still a degree of blame culture that comes with incident investigation. This results in some anxiety among staff involved; however, SEIPS should help with this by shifting the focus from individuals to the whole work systems.

This was a challenging piece of work given the lack of practical training. There are training modules available on SEIPS that the team completed; however, this was lacking in practical application training. Conducting this piece of work has allowed us to connect the theory we learnt as part of the course with the practicalities of conducting a systems thinking-based investigation.

Our next steps in this process are to prepare the report with our results and then evaluate the whole process. Following this we need to roll out training that will incorporate SEIPS/systems thinking to help shift thinking away from the traditional RCA style of investigation.

### Reflections from the Frontline

- Practical examples of how the SEIPS framework is used in healthcare is well documented; however, the practical application on how to get started, what preparation/training is needed and what it could be used for is lacking. This lack of guidance and preparation can become a barrier to implementing the tools.
- Shifting the mindset from a traditional 'linear' way of thinking to a more systems-based approach takes time and effort. It may cause your teams some fear — fear of the unknown and fear that this new approach may not be of any benefit or yield anything extra to the traditional investigation approach.
- Widening the scope of the investigation will allow more contributory factors to be explored and will 'open up' the investigation beyond the specific location of where the event took place, enabling wider collaboration and exploration between different groups. It will allow us to understand others' roles and the expectations from other organisations; for example, from primary and acute care. It is an opportunity to collaborate that we didn't have before.

- Novel communication mechanisms between teams, inside and outside of the care setting, is needed to allow for information to flow and to allow conversations between stakeholders.
- Shifting away from blaming individuals or using human error as the 'root cause' is a huge cultural shift. Balancing accountability of the individual or team with this approach needs careful consideration and a just culture framework needs to be followed.

# References

Anderson, J.E. and Ross, A. (2020). *CAREe QI: A Handbook for Improving Quality through Resilient Systems.* https://resiliencecentre.org.uk/care-qi-handbook/.

Anderson, J.E. and Watt, A.J. (2020). 'Using Safety-II and resilient healthcare principles to learn from never events' in *International Journal for Quality in Health Care,* 00(00), pp. 1–8. Doi: 10.1093/intqhc/mzaa009.

Bowie, P., Jeffcott, S. (2016). 'Human factors and ergonomics for primary care' in *Education Primary Care*, 27(2): pp. 86–93. Doi: 10.1080/14739879.2016.1152658. PMID: 27005836.

Bowie, P. et al. 'Patient safety learning for healthcare improvement: considering the "system context" in medico-legal cases?' in *Journal of Personal Injury Law.* (In Press.)

Carayon, P. et al. (2006). 'Work system design for patient safety: The SEIPS model' in *Quality & Safety in Health Care*, 15(Supplement I), pp. i50–i58.

Donabedian, A. (1966). 'Evaluating the quality of medical care' in *Milbank Memorial Fund Quarterly*, 44(3): pp. 166–206. Doi: 10.2307/3348969.

Hignett, S. et al. (2013). 'State of science: human factors and ergonomics in healthcare' in *Ergonomics*, 56(10): pp. 1491–503. Doi: 10.1080/00140139.2013.822932. PMID: 23926898.

Holden, R.J. et al. (2013). 'SEIPS 2.0: a human factors framework for studying and improving the work of healthcare professionals and patients' in *Ergonomics*, 56(11): pp. 1669–86. Doi: 10.1080/00140139.2013.838643. PMID: 24088063; PMCID: PMC3835697.

Holden, R.J. and Carayon, P. (2021). 'SEIPS 101 and seven simple SEIPS tools' in *BMJ Quality Safety*, 30(11): pp. 901–910. Doi: 10.1136/bmjqs-2020-012538. PMID: 34039748; PMCID: PMC8543199.

Hollnagel, E., Wears, R.L. and Braithwaite, J. (2015). *From Safety-I to Safety-II: A White Paper.* Available at: www.england.nhs.uk/signuptosafety/wp-content/uploads/sites/16/2015/10/safety-1-safety-2-whte-papr.pdf.

Ishikawa K. and Loftus, J.H. (eds.) (1990). *Introduction to quality control.* Tokyo, Japan: 3A Corporation.

Langley, G.J. et al. (2009). *The Improvement Guide. A practical Approach to Enhancing Organizational Performance* (2nd ed). USA: Jossey-bass.

MOD (2015). JSP 912. *Human factors integration for defence systems.* Part 1: Directive. www.gov.uk/government/uploads/system/uploads/attachment_data/file/483176/20150717-JSP_912_Part1_DRU_version_Final-U.pdf.

NHS England (2015). *The Serious Incident Framework.* www.england.nhs.uk/wp-content/uploads/2020/08/serious-incidnt-framwrk.pdf.

NHS Improvement (2018). *Never Events Policy and Framework.* https://www.england.nhs.uk/wp-content/uploads/2020/11/Revised-Never-Events-policy-and-framework-FINAL.pdf.

Russ, A.L. et al. (2013). 'The science of human factors: separating fact from fiction' in *BMJ Quality Safety*, 22(10): pp. 802–8. Doi: 10.1136/bmjqs-2012-001450. PMID: 23592760; PMCID: PMC3786617.

Stanton, N.A. and Young, M.S. (2003). 'Giving ergonomics away? The application of ergonomics methods by novices' in *Applied Ergonomics*, 34(5): pp. 479–90. Doi: 10.1016/S0003-6870(03)00067-X. PMID: 12963333.

Vosper, H., Hignett, S. and Bowie, P. (2018). 'Twelve tips for embedding human factors and ergonomics principles in healthcare education' in *Medical Teach*, 40(4): pp. 357–363. Doi: 10.1080/0142159X.2017.1387240. PMID: 29126356.

WHO (2011). *WHO Patient Safety Curriculum Guide: Multi-professional Edition*. Geneva: World Health Organisation.

Wiig, S., Braithwaite, J. and Clay-Williams, R. (2020). 'It's time to step it up. Why safety investigations in healthcare should look more to safety science' in *International Journal for Quality in Health Care*, *32*(4), pp. 281–284. Doi: 10.1093/intqhc/mzaa013.

Wilson, J.R. (2014). 'Fundamentals of systems ergonomics/human factors' in *Applied Ergonomics*, 45(1), pp. 5–13.

# CHAPTER 4

# Patient and Family Engagement Following Patient Safety Incidents

*Lauren Ramsey, Louise Pye and Jane O'Hara*

## Summary

PSIRF has shifted the policy landscape in multiple ways. Three core changes are the prioritisation of organisational learning, the latitude of learning responses and the explicit focus on compassionate engagement with patients and families.

This chapter explores the key reasons why patient and family engagement following patient safety incidents is important, by introducing the concept of 'compounded harm', as well as emphasising the potential contributions to organisational learning. It also considers what we already know about patient and family engagement and explores some of the ways we might need to look to other sectors, countries and emerging innovations in practice, to learn and improve.

## Background

### Why is Patient and Family Engagement Following Patient Safety Incidents Important?

Rhetoric surrounding the importance of patient and family engagement following patient safety incidents is now well-established in healthcare. Deb Hazeldine illuminates the key reasons why this must consistently translate into practice, from a position of lived experience (Box 4.1).

## BOX 4.1  A Lived Experience Perspective

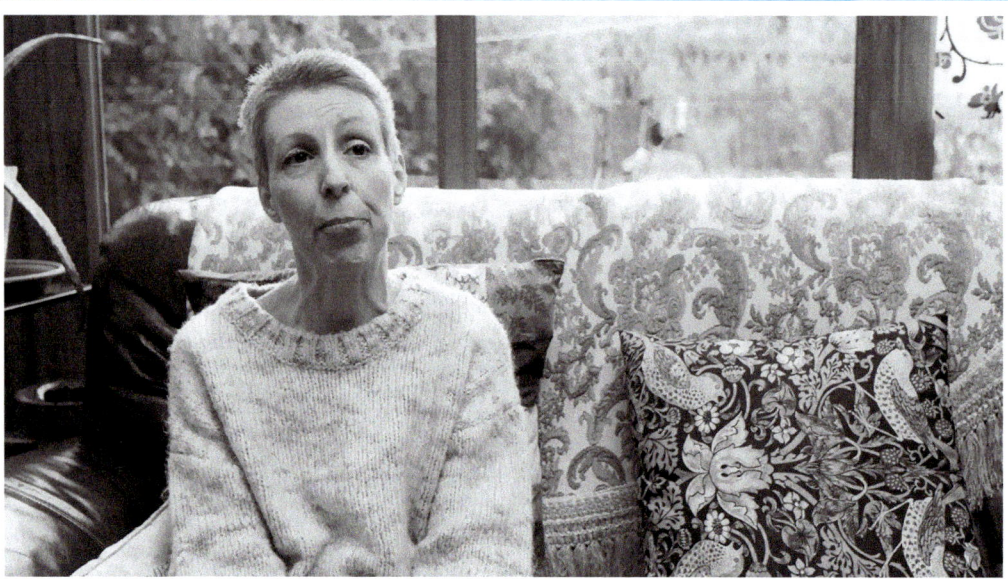

My name is Deb Hazeldine and I became a patient safety campaigner without even knowing it in 2006, when my mum died horrifically in the Mid Staffordshire disaster. She was admitted for physiotherapy, and she died of C. diff. Over many months of trying to complete physiotherapy, she would tell me that she was in pain in her back and in her ribs. And when I raised these concerns, my mum was told that the pain was all in her head and that she just needed to go through the pain barrier and become mobile. It wasn't until after her death, when I read the notes, that I discovered she had preventable falls in hospital, and she had fractures in her back and in her spine. I experienced absolute despair. I just couldn't believe what was happening in front of me. I felt so unable to do anything. I raised concerns and nothing changed. There wasn't an investigation. I didn't for a second think that when my mum had died, when we raised valid concerns, that nothing would be done. We thought instantly, somebody would do something.

My daughter was 12 when my mum died. She was 19 and at university when we sat in London listening to the outcome of a public enquiry which stated some systemic failings. I never thought it would take that many years. The only time I was able to give my mum a voice was many years later when the lead investigator of the Healthcare Commission sat down and said, 'Debra, tell me what happened to your mum'.

I needed someone to say, 'I'm sorry that this happened', and acknowledge that my mum had been failed. When my mum died, I searched and looked for quite some time, but there wasn't anything out there to support the families. There wasn't anywhere where the families had a voice. It always seemed as though it was the system doing something *to* you. It was an investigation that you weren't part of. I couldn't quite understand how your most dearest loved one wasn't having a voice. You weren't there, actually sitting at the table. With my own mum's death, nobody had asked my opinion for many, many years.

For me, knowledge is power. And if you don't share that, we can't ask questions about processes that we don't understand, that we don't know, that we're not involved in. And

> I've found over the years, families desperately want a voice. They want to be able to say, 'This was my loved one. This is our family member. Can we please be involved?' Honesty, transparency and candour would have changed my life dramatically.
>
> *Deb Hazeldine MBE, Patient safety campaigner following the death of her mum in Mid Staffordshire Hospital in 2006. You can access a video where Deb speaks about the importance of patient and family involvement in more detail at learn-together.org.uk.*

## Meeting the Needs of Patients and Families Following Patient Safety Incidents — A Moral Duty?

In basic terms, what patients and families most need following something going wrong in healthcare has been known for the last two decades (e.g. Bismark and Paterson, 2005). These needs are often wide-ranging and specific to individual circumstances; however, at the crux of it are human beings, relationships between them, and the physical, emotional and/or financial impacts they are experiencing. Broad themes have been described across a multitude of papers that span a range of literatures (e.g. open disclosure (Harrison et al., 2017; Iedema et al., 2008), communication resolution programmes (Mello et al., 2020) and reasons for medico-legal action (Bismark and Dauer, 2006)). They have also been outlined in a recent review (Ramsey et al., 2022) and can be summarised as the needs for:

- Acknowledgement and apology
- Their views to be listened to and valued
- Answers to their questions
- A coherent account of what happened and why
- Clear expectations and timelines
- Relevant practical and emotional support
- System change to prevent future harm
- Compensation (where necessary)

Where these needs are not met, this can feel at odds with basic expectations of what caring organisations are set up to do. Bismark and Paterson (2005) made a compelling argument to suggest that, actually, there is a need to go back to basics in healthcare and warrant these human experiences with a human response. Therefore, it could be argued that meeting these needs is a *moral duty* of health services and the various agencies that support them within the policy and regulatory landscape.

Understanding and acknowledging this moral duty has emerged slowly over the past two decades. In 2009, the Being Open Framework was launched, followed by the Duty of Candour becoming enshrined in legislation in 2014. It also aligns with the three strategic aims — insight, involvement and improvement, outlined within the NHS Patient Safety Strategy launched in 2019. Further, the right to an apology, support through an investigation regarding any complaint of poor quality or unsafe care, and the commitment to learn from any complaint or investigation and improve services in response to that learning, are now explicitly written into the *NHS Constitution for England* (2021). In some ways, this *moral duty* to support people after healthcare harm could be regarded as a simple extension of the *duty of care* of services to patients and families experienced before healthcare harm. In short, the same concepts applied to healthcare provision should remain in the aftermath of something going wrong.

## The importance of the Patient and Family Perspective to Support Organisational Learning

In addition to this moral duty, there are also very logical reasons for involving patients and families in organisational learning activities following patient safety incidents. It has long been established in scientific literature that patients and families can reliably share important information about risk and the safety of care (O'Hara *et al.*, 2018; Etchegaray *et al.*, 2016; Iedema *et al.*, 2012; Weissman *et al.*, 2008; Weingart *et al.*, 2005). It is recognised that this source of safety information extends beyond what is written in medical notes, or what healthcare staff are able to share, and provides valuable opportunities for organisational learning. This is perhaps unsurprising as patients and families tend to be the only consistent component of their whole healthcare journey, sometimes spanning multiple services and care providers, and over long periods of time. People are also increasingly managing their own care in the home and in community settings. This evidence helped to inform calls made from Vincent *et al.* (2017) to look at the 'evolution of patient journeys in much greater depth and assume that patients and families will be partners in investigations'.

By not engaging with patients and families when something has gone wrong, services not only fail in their moral duty but also omit a valuable source of information that might help them understand what happened and why, impacting opportunities to learn and improve. Failing to meet the needs of patients and families following safety incidents, and their experience of the processes that follow, can also lead to further, and sometimes significant, harm. This has been termed 'compounded harm'.

## What is Compounded Harm?

Compounded harm is a concept that defines harm not caused by the patient safety incident itself, but, rather, the harm caused by the processes that follow (Wailling *et al.*, 2022). Although it may not be possible to eliminate patient safety incidents entirely, what is possible is to proceed in ways that dignify their experience and do not result in additional trauma.

One common misconception is that the act of engaging the patient and their family can itself re-traumatise them and, therefore. should be avoided or be 'light touch'. It is, of course, very important to recognise and be sensitive to grief or trauma and adapt means of communication and timings accordingly; however, avoiding engagement entirely, or failing to confront what happened, goes against evidence that suggests that, actually, patient and family involvement has the potential to alleviate some of the trauma caused by the original incident and go some way to rebuilding trust.

In a report from the Parliamentary and Health Service Ombudsman (PHSO, 2023), analysis of 22 cases of NHS complaint investigations involving avoidable death identified several factors that contributed to compounded harm:

- A failure to be honest when things go wrong
- A lack of support to navigate systems after an incident
- Poor quality investigations
- A failure to respond to complaints in a timely and compassionate way
- Inadequate apologies
- Unsatisfactory learning responses

These findings led to recommendations in two core areas. First, accountability for a robust and compassionate response to harm, which supports learning for systems and healing for families. Second, evidencing that patient safety is a top Government and NHS priority.

In summary, patient and family engagement following patient safety incidents is important for three foundational reasons. First, it meets a moral duty of health services that can contribute to restoration and healing. Second, the valuable perspective of patients and families can enhance the breadth and depth of learning opportunities that may be otherwise missed. Third, it reduces the risk of patients and families experiencing compounded harm.

# What do We Already Know About Patient and Family Engagement Following Patient Safety Incidents?

Patient and family engagement and involvement following patient safety incidents means different things to different people. It is perhaps useful to consider it in terms of three separate concepts; however, even within these concepts there is disagreement and variation. We present a summary of each concept below.

## Concept 1: What Does Family Mean?

In cases where it is not possible to involve the patient (e.g. where the incident has led to a death) or where an individual wishes for support from others close to them, family may be involved. Sometimes termed next of kin or an emergency contact, there is no legal basis or clear rules surrounding who could or should be involved. Family may mean anyone who has a direct and close relationship to the patient, including but not limited to that person's spouse, adopted family member, their closest living blood relative or a friend.

## Concept 2: What Does Safety Incident Mean?

Patient safety incidents are any unintended or unexpected incident which could have, or did, lead to harm for one or more patients receiving healthcare. The rationale for identifying and reporting patient safety incidents is to support health services to learn from mistakes and to take action to reduce the likelihood of recurrence.

## Concept 3: What Does Engagement and Involvement Mean?

Often, *engagement* and *involvement* are terms used interchangeably. However, PSIRF makes an important distinction between the two. This is because PSIRF sets out a number of learning response types that healthcare organisations in England can draw upon, only some of which offer opportunities for involvement, but all of which should be underpinned by engagement.

Engagement is a general term that refers to everything organisations do to communicate and work with patients and their families within the processes that follow a patient safety incident. For example, disclosing the incident through the Duty of Candour, providing an apology and explaining what will happen next. Irrespective of the incident response type used according to PSIRF, and regardless of whether the patient or family chooses to be involved in the investigation or not, staff should always seek to engage (Figure 4.1).

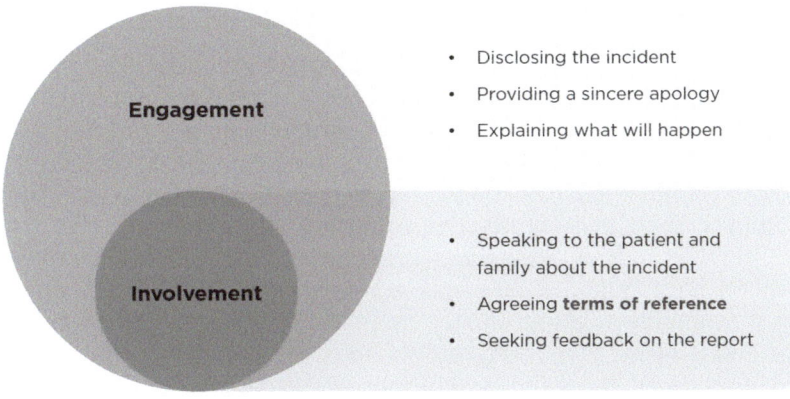

**Figure 4.1** Relationship Between Engagement and Involvement. (Reproduced with permission — Learn Together Investigation Guide accessed via learn-together.org.uk.)

However, involvement is a more specific term that refers to activity relating to supporting the explicit investigation aims. For example, understanding what happened from the patient and family perspective to support learning and seeking feedback on a draft version of the investigation report. Involvement opportunities such as these may only be appropriate for certain response types (e.g. PSIIs).

## A Patient and Family Perspective

From the perspective of patients and families, the incident and how it is handled by the health service can lead them to distrust services and staff more generally, which is important to rebuild over time. Particularly, for those who may need to use health services for ongoing treatment and care and for those who will need to access health services in the future. Evidence indicates that patient and family engagement, when done well, can go some way to restoring faith in the healthcare system and contribute to reconciliation following a traumatic event (McQueen et al., 2022), as well as reducing the likelihood of litigation. Nonetheless, desire and capacity to be involved from the patient and family inevitably varies, and some choose not to be involved temporarily or permanently, for many known and unknown reasons. Involvement must be optional; however, it is important to leave the door open to involvement, if and when the circumstances feel right for the patient or family, which may extend beyond the typical organisational timelines of a response.

A further issue is the sparsity of approaches that are truly equitable and inclusive. This means that safety inequities are twofold. For example, people with learning disabilities are more likely to be affected by patient safety incidents (Louch et al., 2021), yet systemic safety inequities may mean that they are least likely to be able to engage in an organisational response (Ramsey et al., 2022b). To avoid exacerbating existing healthcare inequities, it is crucial that health services aim to make sure that engagement and involvement is accessible and inclusive to all. This means adapting to suit different people where possible, rather than expecting people to adapt to suit the health service.

One example of where this has been attempted is the Healthcare Safety Investigation Branch (HSIB) Family Inclusivity Toolkit, which focuses on three key areas: the communication needs, the health and well-being needs, and the social and community needs of families, to enable investigators to provide tailored support (HSIB, 2020). When first engaging with families, investigators are encouraged to ask specific questions to those affected. In these conversations it is hoped that individuals will be asked what approach works best for them to ensure they are heard and to ensure the organisational approach is inclusive. Some of the needs identified may be long standing and require some form of adjustment in approach, whereas other needs may be specific to the safety incident that has occurred. Whatever the need, identifying the right approach in partnership ensures that the opportunities of involvement are maximised.

## A Clinician's Perspective

From the perspective of clinical healthcare staff, evidence suggests that most believe that patient and family involvement has the potential to enhance the quality of incident responses, promote an open culture and contribute to organisational learning and improvement. However, culturally engrained fears surrounding involvement are difficult to overcome. Challenges in practice include absent multidisciplinary input, unmanageable workloads, high staff turnover, inadequate training and lack of support. There is also the need to consider the fears surrounding litigation and the complexities this adds. For example, staff report concerns of inadequate legal protection, being blamed for systems failures and managing conflicting information surrounding the implications of apology. To help to overcome common myths and fears, the Scottish Public Services Ombudsmen produced a guide focused on how to make a good apology (2020).

## An Engagement Lead's Perspective

Engagement lead is a term used to define people who lead on engaging with, and involving those affected by a patient safety incident. In an attempt to meet the needs of patients and families (see above), healthcare organisations may adopt a range of different models to employ engagement leads locally, informed by various contextual factors (e.g. size of the organisation, staffing levels, available resource, underpinning rationale for responding to incidents). In the three examples that follow, three models for engagement lead roles are described.

*Investigating as a role* Organisations may employ staff whose role is purely focused on responding to patient safety incidents and engaging with patients and families. This work may be conducted by teams of varying sizes who operate in various ways. For example, they may work during usual working hours Monday to Friday, they may work flexibly or may be resourced seven days a week. These staff may also work to respond to any patient safety incident across the Trust or may work within a particular service or clinical area. They may work alone or in partnership with others in a similar or a different role. For example, Trusts may use a 'buddy-system', which aims to combine the skills and insights of an engagement expert and a clinical expert. In addition, organisations may employ bank staff who have specific skills, experience or expertise, on a long-term basis, or call upon them during periods of high demand or when experiencing staffing issues. Box 4.2 highlights the experience of investigating as a role.

---

**BOX 4.2    Experiences of Investigating as a Role**

'Involving patients and families in an investigation is the right thing to do. I have found their perspective on events and their observations about potential improvements invaluable for producing a comprehensive report with meaningful recommendations. Such outcomes are important for organisational improvement. But for the family, the investigation is about so much more. The investigator has a significant responsibility to them.

As an incident investigator the benefits of having dedicated time for the review and being able to work flexibly to be responsive to family needs, lends itself to a better experience for all parties. I used the Learn Together guides (learn-together.org.uk) which helped enormously in providing a framework to maximise the quality of "when and what" information is shared; and most importantly to guide families at what is already a difficult time. Any investigator, whether new or experienced, will find the investigator guide invaluable.

When it comes to family engagement the role of the investigator is rewarding; never more so than when you have fruitful and supportive conversations with families and provide them with answers to their questions. One family involved in the study commented "We just wanted to start out by thanking you for your professionalism and fairness in handling the investigation. At all times we have felt supported and well informed, and we do appreciate that".

Equally the role can be extremely challenging. From a practical perspective, more frequent engagement provides opportunities to raise more questions. This is not a bad thing but may pose challenges if outside the investigation terms of reference. Investigation timeframes (under the Serious Incident Framework) set an endpoint that was not necessarily conducive to involving families who, for various reasons, postponed conversations or did not get around to reading report drafts. In addition, trying to produce an approved clinically accurate draft report for family review within the timeframes posed a different set of logistical challenges. These challenges should not exist under the new incident framework.

The role can also be emotionally distressing. With greater engagement there is a risk of increasing negative consequences. You get to better know the family — you feel their anguish. You try to do your best for families but may unintentionally compound their harm with a misjudged comment. There may be differences in opinion about assigning blame or in understanding where "best practice" may be different to what the family see as "practice that is best". The need for empathic communication skills cannot be underestimated.

The Learn Together documentation helps to set the landscape and expectations and guide investigators and families through the investigation to optimise the outcome and the experiences whilst getting there.'

*Jacqui Evans, York & Scarborough Teaching Hospitals NHS Foundation Trust*

*Investigating as part of another role*   Another frequently used model for organisations is to add the responsibility of responding to incidents to the work plans of existing staff working in separate roles, such as patient safety, governance, quality improvement or frontline clinical staff. There may be some benefits of this model, including providing clinical staff with additional role responsibility or career development; supporting clinical input into investigations; and not requiring organisations to find extra resources for investigations. However, it can equally be argued that this model comes with some associated problems. For example, without protected time and space, as well as adequate training and support, it is possible that these staff may lack the specialised knowledge, skills and resources required to meaningfully engage with patients and families in ways that do not compound harm.

*The Patient and Family Liaison Officer role*   The Patient and Family Liaison Officer (PFLO) role (often referred to as Family Liaison Officer (FLO)) is becoming increasingly established in healthcare. In this role, staff are specifically employed to support the patient and family engagement aspect of incident responses. For those organisations who adopt this model, there may be an individual fulfilling this duty or it may involve multiple staff. The remit of the PFLO may differ, as well as the extent they are embedded within the wider patient safety team. For example, a PFLO may only be responsible for working on cases of severe harm or death, where families are keen to be involved and/or incidents relating to particular services. Their work may also involve investigating, or they may work in collaboration with investigators, in which case their perception of autonomy and agency may differ and require multidisciplinary buy-in across the wider organisation for the family voice to be truly heard and valued. See Box 4.3 for an evaluation of the PFLO role.

### BOX 4.3   An Evaluation of the Patient and Family Liaison Officer (PFLO) Role

'In August 2019, in response to local learning around engagement with patients and families and national policy and guidance, the Corporate Patient Safety Team at Nottingham University Hospitals appointed a PFLO. A key focus of the role was to support patients, families, and carers throughout incident investigations, particularly during the Trust's Serious Incident (SI) and Learning from Deaths processes. A rapid formative process evaluation of the implementation of the PFLO was undertaken between September and December 2020. Fifteen key Trust stakeholders participated in qualitative video or face to face interviews during September and October 2020. Semi-structured interviews were designed to explore stakeholder perspectives on implementation and engagement with the PFLO role.

The evaluation found that gaining executive support for the PFLO role was vital. To develop the role, the Corporate Patient Safety Team drew upon internal and external reports and guidance, and liaised with other Trusts and an external expert in patient and family liaison in the context of investigations in the NHS. At the role planning stage, the different layers to the scope and remit of the role were recognised. This included supporting families through a serious incident investigation and hearing their voice in the investigation. In the planning stages, the importance of communication skills and interaction with families and staff involved in the serious incident investigation process was also recognised.

The evaluation found that the role had to integrate into the established working practices of staff engaged in the serious incident investigation process and specialist services that delivered a model of patient and family liaison. As such, ways of working required some degree of adjustment. Participants considered that prior communication of the remit, priorities and capability of the role would have helped to understand how the role was to become part of their processes.

The notion of the role acting as a bridge between families and the Trust can be a useful way of describing how participants interpreted the role. To act as a bridge required skill on the part of the PFLO and was achieved by keeping information flowing between all parties involved and, taking care to be clear that the serious incident process for the Trust is about learning and not apportioning blame. However, family liaison in the context of a serious incident investigation is also about the healing process for a family. The complexity of striking a balance between the right level of involvement for a family, and what the formal organisational process is trying to achieve, was acknowledged. The role being corporate brought a sense of independence from the divisions. This was seen to reduce bias and increase objectivity. The role was interpreted as being able to act both as an advocate for the family, but also as a representative of the hospital.

The evaluation found that, as a result of competing clinical pressures (despite the best intentions of the panel), regularly contacting the family, appreciating their concerns and providing timely responses in a way that meets their emotional needs can be a difficult goal to achieve. Participants felt that the PFLO's experience and approach meant that families were supported to work through what they wanted and needed to say prior to meetings and after meetings. The relationship enabled the role to brief panel members on how the family were feeling and on any family dynamics. From panel members' perspectives this feedback enabled them to approach meetings with a level of insight and awareness and was interpreted as providing a strong foundation for face-to-face meetings.

The evaluation found that from the perspective of staff, support for families from the role was considered to be invaluable. A key factor was consistent and regular contact to provide information on the serious incident investigation process and progress updates. This was interpreted as taking pressure off families by having somebody passing information back to the investigating panel. Participants considered that through acting as a liaison between families and the organisation, the role empowered families by giving them choice in how they were communicated with, as well as giving them the opportunity to have their voice heard in the investigation.

Creating boundaries around the PFLO offer was complex. In some cases, the role could be involved with families until the coroner's inquest and beyond. This means that the role may extend for a year or more, involving the families and multiple stakeholders. Participants questioned what emotional support the role received. The emotional burden of dealing with a multitude of cases simultaneously (including both adults and children), was recognised.'

*Dr Charlotte Overton, Research Fellow within the Safer Systems, Cultures and Practices theme of the Yorkshire and Humber Patient Safety Research Collaboration*

What is clear is that there is no one perfect organisational model. Rather, each comes with a set of benefits and challenges which must be balanced and considered in light of local organisational context. Rather than the role of individuals fulfilling the duty of patient and family engagement, these decisions should be grounded in the ability to meet their needs, as well as the needs of other key stakeholders. Regardless of the organisational model opted for, the responsibility of patient and family engagement should also be recognised as part of a professional and skilled role, with protected time and space, underpinned by relevant training and support.

## The Impact of Litigation

Evidence from NHS Resolution (2018) suggests that patients and families who pursued litigation were often not invited to discuss the findings of any local investigation. They also reported inadequate or inappropriate apology and explanation of events, unsatisfactory written and verbal communication, and feelings that no meaningful outcome had been achieved. This is despite guidance from NHS resolution based on 'The Compensation Act 2006' stating that 'An apology, an offer of treatment or other redress, shall not of itself amount to an admission of negligence or breach of statutory duty'. This aligns with other evidence suggesting that patients and families who felt involved in transparent investigation processes reported being less likely to pursue litigation, whereas others felt the need to fight for progress, using methods such as threatening litigation (Bell *et al.*, 2012).

## The Impact of the Healthcare Setting

The needs of patients and families following patient safety incidents have overarching similarities across healthcare settings. However, there are important differences. Understanding these nuances can help organisations know how to undertake involvement and engagement in ways that are inclusive and appropriate.

Examples of issues experienced across different healthcare settings include:

- **Maternity care** — for example, situations where mother and baby are not able to be cared for together due to different medical interventions required.
- **Paediatrics** — for example, the need to speak with the child, but also to involve those with parental responsibility.
- **Mental health** — for example, not being able to speak to the person affected due to their capacity to understand information and make decisions.
- **Prison healthcare** — for example, those in custody may consider those they share accommodation with to be family, rather than those external to the prison system.
- **Community care** — for example, a suicide that happens in the community setting and the individual has a limited history of interaction with the service responsible for responding.
- **Multi-agency healthcare** — for example, a complex unexplained death following a history of mental and physical health symptoms cared for in primary, secondary, tertiary and community settings.

## Learn Together

A programme of research called Learn Together (www.learn-together.org.uk) found that some of the foundational constraints were more pronounced or differed between healthcare settings. The complexities listed below were apparent in acute care, but often appeared more common and complex in mental healthcare. This was thought to be largely due to the nature of incidents being investigated, which often involved suspected death by suicide among other severe harm incidents.

*Sourcing the appropriate next of kin details*   Following a death, finding the right person or people to involve often felt like an informal investigation in and of itself. Investigators were often required to liaise with different services, care teams and the coroner's office to piece together potentially incomplete, outdated and/or conflicting information. Some felt uncomfortable making forced and difficult decisions based on limited information. In the meantime, the investigation had sometimes progressed without inviting involvement, or there were significant delays in anticipation of it. The most appropriate next of kin was also sometimes difficult to pinpoint for a variety of reasons such as confidentiality dilemmas. Examples include where the service user made explicit requests to not involve family in their care or where family were unaware the individual was receiving mental health care. Additionally, staff often had to navigate complex family dynamics, such as fractious relationships and histories of abuse and domestic violence, which sometimes contributed to the reasons services users had needed to receive mental healthcare. Other issues included commonly missing or outdated next of kin information on NHS Trust systems, elderly or otherwise vulnerable next of kin, and multiple people wanting to be the main point of contact on behalf of the family.

*Juggling the ethical dilemma of involving and re-traumatising*   Particularly in instances of severe harm or death across settings, staff felt responsible for juggling the ethical dilemma of inviting involvement, but also not wanting to overburden or re-traumatise those who did not want to or did not feel able to be involved. Both mental health Trusts involved in the Learn Together research programme had a history of an opt-in approach to involvement. In practice, this meant that a single letter was sent providing follow-up contact information and in cases of no follow-up, it was assumed that families had made an informed choice to not be involved. Instead, in some instances, this meant that they had not received the invitation, they were unable to comprehend the invitation to be involved at a difficult time in their lives, they did not trust that the organisation would listen to their views if they did become involved, or they did not want to be involved temporarily to allow for grieving and recuperation. Interestingly, one of the mental health Trusts transitioned to an opt-out approach and saw an increase in involvement. This choice was prompted by families asking to be involved on receiving the investigation report, often via the coroner. Some felt that finding out information for the first time via the coroner indicated that the organisation did not care, nor wanted to learn from what had happened. Although the move to an opt-out approach to involvement was considered largely positive, the same Trust reflected on an experience of involving a next of kin who was a mental health service user who later made a suicide attempt as a result of being involved in an investigation. The responsibility of juggling this ethical dilemma was a significant part of the role as an investigator across settings.

*Fluctuating involvement*   The involvement of patients and families across settings naturally fluctuated throughout the course of an investigation and was rarely consistent, even for those who were most enthusiastically involved initially. Some openly spoke about the reasons that their involvement would fluctuate upfront, such as needing to step back to preserve their emotional energy and look after their own needs, or managing other simultaneous processes such as litigation, complaints or inquest. Others decided to step back when they felt that the investigation had served its purpose or no longer met their needs. However, in many cases, investigators were left to make sense of the reasons that involvement might have fluctuated and decide how to proceed based upon those assumptions. Some investigators referred to feeling disheartened or frustrated at unrequited attempts to engage. In mental healthcare, particularly in cases of suspected death by suicide, additional complexities include family self-blame or shame; cultural or religious reasons to not engage in investigations of suicide; the complexity of a history of mental health issues in the family and chaotic family lifestyles.

*Scale of the incident and potential for learning* In cases of suspected death by suicide in mental healthcare, next of kin were often raising more fundamental issues, spanning multiple care providers and external agents, and reflecting on issues over a relatively long period of time. Adding further nuance were suicides completed in the community, and where service users had limited interaction with the organisation responsible for responding. This meant that the often-limited terms of reference regarding the scale and scope of the investigation did not cohere with the families' experience, what they felt needed to be investigated and what they would like to see improved. This sometimes resulted in an additional layer of frustration for families who sensed that their involvement was futile. Involving families sooner, setting clear expectations and having flexible terms of reference was perceived to help, but, for some, the investigation system felt like it was against the very thing that they wanted the investigation to achieve. In acute care settings, investigations were generally more focused and discrete. For instance, in maternity, although investigations were often complex, the length of time the investigation covered tended to be limited to the pregnancy journey, or in cases of surgical complication, the web of contributory factors was relatively clearer and less nuanced than a suspected death by suicide.

*Emotional labour for staff leading investigations* The emotional labour undertaken by investigators throughout the course of an investigation was evident across settings. Investigators were often placed in the difficult position of making contact with patients and families who had varied experiences of care; being the first port of call for their questions and frustrations; and navigating systemic barriers to do what felt like the 'right thing'. Investigators also reflected on hearing multiple perspectives which were often at odds, and being responsible for making a judgement about the weighting of perspectives and what the final report should include. One investigator likened the report to a piece of pottery which multiple people have tried to shape, and another reflected on their efforts often feeling like a thankless task when nobody was happy with the report at the end of it. Due to the nature of death and suicide being the topic of investigations in mental healthcare, this may be particularly difficult for investigators and was the reasons for some staff turnover during the programme of research. Additionally, a mental health patient safety manager referred to giving her team of investigators a rest by working on complaints, instead of investigations of suicide.

## System-Level Challenges

The introduction of PSIRF creates the opportunity for greater freedom and flexibility in incident investigation management. Nevertheless, there are few resources available currently to support patient safety leaders to practically apply these new approaches for learning, action and improvement. Other concerns include the risk of healthcare inequities being exacerbated, patients and families escalating incidents that are no longer being investigated in other ways, such as complaints and litigation, and the risk that organisations with poor culture do not carry out investigations when there are opportunities to learn. It has also been argued that learning opportunities are not self-evident until the investigation is complete; therefore, determining on that basis is challenging.

Although key stakeholders are generally in agreement that patient and family engagement is something that health services *should* be doing, there are various tensions and challenges in practice that need to be balanced, particularly as the needs of different stakeholders diverge.

Here are some examples:

- PSIRF asks healthcare organisations in England to prioritise organisational learning, and to do so by deciding which incidents to investigate based on potential for learning. Although this may meet ambitions for learning, it may be counter to the needs of the patients and families whose priority is often to fully understand what happened and the preventability of

their specific case. In short, different stakeholders might have different priorities for deciding what warrants an investigation.
- In efforts to protect staff and support a just culture, organisations may not facilitate the coming together of patients and families who have been affected by a patient safety incident with those directly responsible for care. However, evidence suggests that for some staff in some circumstances, this may actually contribute to their secondary harm and deny them the opportunity to heal, similar to the experiences of patients and families who feel that coming together to discuss what happened within a supported, facilitated meeting, might be therapeutic.

In this section, we have introduced some key concepts within, and challenges for, engagement and involvement of patients and families in processes that follow patient safety incidents. It is important to understand the difference between engagement and involvement activity and to be clear that engagement *is always advised* even when patients and families do not necessarily wish to *be actively involved* in incident responses. There is no one way to engage and involve families, and organisations need to understand how different settings might create different needs and expectations. The policy landscape will both create and address different challenges for engagement and involvement, and services would be advised to look to a variety of models and undertake regular evaluation of whatever model they adopt.

# What Could Patient and Family Engagement Following Patient Safety Incidents Look Like in the Future?

## What Can We Learn from Other Sectors?

Healthcare has often looked to other sectors to understand how to improve patient safety. Interestingly, engagement and involvement has been one area of healthcare where other sectors or settings have had less influence. However, across all industries and sectors, when an event occurs and a form of investigation is needed to understand what happened, whether it is for purposes of learning or to establish culpability, a system is required to plan for how people within that response are communicated with.

The police force undertakes one of the largest areas of investigative work. Police respond to various reported incidents ranging from public order events, injuries on our roads, minor crimes and serious and complex crimes where serious injury or death occurs. However, alongside such investigations is a recognition of the important role of supporting victims and witnesses of such incidents throughout the criminal justice process.

The police force has an explicit set of expectations for those who are affected by a crime, and these are enshrined in their Code of Practice (2020) for Victims of Crime in England and Wales. This code sets out the services and a minimum standard that must be provided to victims of crime by organisations (referred to as service providers) in England and Wales. This code describes what a 'victim' is, and who this term refers to, before outlining a series of rights that they have within the process of an investigation, including the right to be able to understand and to be understood; to have the details of the crime recorded without unjustified delay; to be provided with information when reporting the crime; to be referred to services that support victims and have services and support tailored to your needs; and to be provided with information about compensation.

Victims of crime also have the right to make a victim personal statement where they can share how they have been affected by what has happened so that others can understand the impact of the situation. Accomplishing these rights of individuals are the responsibilities for anyone responding to a crime, but in certain situations a specific role of a Family Liaison Officer (FLO) is used. The role of a FLO is to gather evidence and information from the family, and to sensitively provide support and information to them in certain types of crime.

In transport, A Memorandum of Understanding (MoU) has been established between the Chief Inspectors of the UK Air, Marine and Rail Accident Investigation Branches (the AIBs), and the National Police Chiefs' Council (NPCC) to detail how effective investigations of transport accidents and any crime associated with them are conducted. These investigations would run in parallel and would be independent of each other. However, those affected need to be considered by all parties to ensure 'an effective dialogue with families'.

The Prisons and Probation Ombudsman conducts independent investigations with the aim to make custody and community supervision safer and fairer. These investigations provide families or next of kin with a point of contact to act as a conduit between them and the investigation process. This FLO role will be a family or next of kin's main point of contact for all questions and information sharing.

Established in 2017, the Healthcare Safety Investigation Branch (HSIB)[1] aims to conduct independent investigations into NHS funded care in England. HSIB defines family engagement as 'the prompt, effective liaison between a family and an investigation to ensure the family is integral to the investigation and is treated professionally, respectfully and according to their individual needs'. This definition is adapted from the, then named, National Policing Improvement Agency (NPIA) family liaison guidance (National Policing Improvement Agency, 2008).

This liaison is conducted by trained investigators who are the central point of contact for patients and families. Through a model of family engagement these investigators ensure that patients and their families are central to the investigation processes; the differing needs of individuals are recognised; the support required to be part of the investigation is provided; and information about additional support is provided where necessary. It is the espoused view of HSIB that meaningful engagement with families throughout the investigation process can support the production of high-quality reports and an improved experience of the investigation for all involved.

## An International Perspective

Patient and family engagement following patient safety incidents is a global healthcare concern. There is a growing portfolio of research and service development internationally, including an exploration of hospital manager and investigators' experience of patient and family engagement in the Netherlands (Kok *et al.*, 2018) and the formation of the Patient Engagement Action Team in Canada (2018). Various interventions designed to support patient and family engagement have also been tested in the USA, including communication resolution programmes (Mello *et al.*, 2020; Moore and Mello, 2017; Mello *et al.*, 2016; Mello *et al.*, 2014), the disclosure, apology and offer model (Bell *et al.*, 2012) and the Improving Post-Event Analysis and Communication Together (IMPACT) tool (Ottosen *et al.*, 2016) as well as the development of a model focused on using compassionate communication skills when involving patients and families in NHS Scotland (McQueen *et al.*, 2022). Box 4.4 shows a case study from Norway.

---

1 Healthcare Safety Investigation Branch (HSIB) was formed in 2017 and was funded by the Department of Health and Social Care. HSIB carried out independent safety investigations into NHS-funded care across England through two programmes: national investigations and maternity investigations. After the Health and Care Act 2022 was passed, between April 2022 and October 2023 HSIB went through a period of transformation. The HSIB maternity investigations programme is now hosted by the Care Quality Commission and is known as the Maternity and Newborn Safety Investigations (MNSI) programme. The national investigations programme has continued under Health Services Safety Investigations Body (HSSIB)

## BOX 4.4   Learning from Norway

'Despite patient and family involvement being recognised as a key contributor to the international quality and safety agenda, Norway has struggled to establish it within regulatory practice. However, the Norwegian Board of Health Supervision responded to heavy critique by establishing new involvement strategy and a program for user involvement in regulation which included funding of development projects within regulatory bodies across Norway to improve user involvement in regulatory practice. One of these projects was developing a new method to specifically improve involvement of next of kin in regulatory practice after a patient had died in an adverse event (Wiig et al., 2021a,b; Wigg et al., 2020). Collaboratively, with colleagues from the University of Stavanger, we conducted an independent process evaluation of the new regulatory method and explored the perspectives of both regulators and next of kin experiences based on learning from families of patient deaths. The method involved a preparatory meeting between regulatory inspectors (medical doctor and legal practitioner), a two-hour face to face meeting with next of kin who had lost a close family member in a fatal adverse event to discuss issues relating to the incident, and the offer of follow-up support.

From the perspective of next of kin, involvement was a largely positive experience. Next of kin wanted to be involved, they were able to provide in-depth knowledge about the adverse event and the healthcare system, and involvement meant much more than simply sharing information, as it also had therapeutic effects and contributed to trust building. A defining factor of the positive experience was the individual inspectors' professional, social and human skills.

Next of kin did, however, experience challenges, including emotional aspects of involvement and difficulties understanding the regulators' role. There was also a suggestion to strengthen available information about involvement and the investigation process for next of kin.

From the perspective of the inspectors, again, positive experiences were highlighted, including the ability of next of kin involvement to inform the investigation and the emotionally challenging nature being in accordance with political expectation.

Nevertheless, negative experiences included increasing the workload of regulators, and involvement challenging the principles of equal treatment. There was also a suggestion to improve selection criteria and allow differentiation.

Although next of kin involvement was emotionally challenging from both perspectives, increased regulators' workload and there were calls to strengthen the approach, experiences were largely positive, both in terms of the contribution to improving the investigation and therapeutically. The Norwegian healthcare system has demonstrated that there is significant potential for involvement; however, there is a need for co-designing the investigation process, as well as more guidance and research focused on what constitutes effective involvement, and increased awareness amongst wide-ranging stakeholders.'

*Professor Siri Wiig, Centre Director and Professor of Quality and Safety in Healthcare Systems, University of Stavanger*

## Innovations in Engagement

As well as learning from other sectors and healthcare agencies, there are a number of important innovations that are shaping how patients and families are engaged and involved during incident responses.

**56** Patient Safety: Emerging Applications of Safety Science

*The Learn Together programme* Commencing in 2019, this programme of research aimed to develop and test new guidance for involving and engaging families in incident investigations. Importantly, this research employed 'co-design' methods throughout the research, meaning that everything was developed with patient and family representatives, engagement leads, managers, healthcare staff, policy makers and other important stakeholders. In 2023, this research produced the final versions of materials to support (i) patients and families to be involved and engaged in PSIIs; and (ii) investigators to involve and engage patients and families in PSIIs. These materials have been tested on real investigations within health services and redesigned based on evidence generated. They are designed to complement each other, and support both engagement leads and patients and families through the same five-stage process (Figure 4.2).

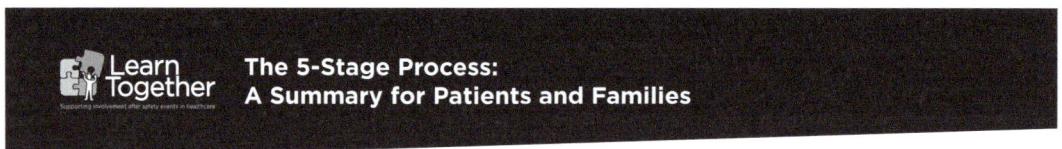

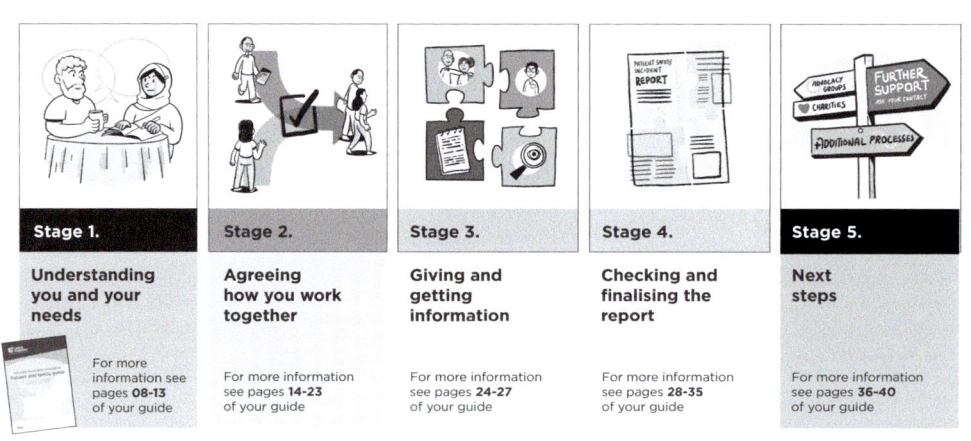

© Copyright Bradford Teaching Hospitals NHS Foundation Trust, 2023. All rights reserved. This material must not be reproduced or shared without permission from Professor Jane O'Hara (yqsradmin@bthft.nhs.uk)

**Figure 4.2** The Learn Together Five-Stage Process. (Reproduced with permission.)

The Five-Stage Process has been designed to support organisations and engagement leads to undertake PSIIs, in ways that *reduce compounded harm*. You can explore all the evidence from the programme and the materials, including a series of supporting videos, on the programme website: learn-together.org.uk. The evidence generated from the Learn Together programme has been incorporated into PSIRF.

## Patient and Family Advocacy

In December 2020, following an extensive exploration of reports of poor maternity care and outcomes at Shrewsbury and Telford Hospital NHS Trust, Donna Ockenden published her first report alongside a number of urgent actions for maternity services across England to address. Among these actions were two relating to the need to listen to women and families (Ockenden, 2020):

- Trusts must create an independent senior advocate role which reports to both the Trust and the Local Maternity Systems Boards.
- The advocate must be available to families attending follow-up meetings with clinicians where concerns about maternity or neonatal care are discussed, particularly where there has been an adverse outcome.

These actions have been embraced by NHS England and the role of maternity and neonatal independent senior advocate has been created. This has a defined job description and there is a requirement for all advocates to undergo training. This role, and the training for advocates, is currently being piloted within maternity services across England.

*Restorative approaches*   Interest is growing internationally about how healthcare services might respond differently to patient safety incidents and healthcare harm. This different way of responding can be loosely termed 'restorative approaches'. This way of responding in some way subverts the traditional approach to patient safety incident classification and investigation driven by organisational needs (which prioritises learning) and replaces it with one driven by the needs of those involved and affected by patient safety events.

A working definition of a 'restorative approach' has been proposed (Wailling *et al.*, 2022):

'A voluntary, relational process where all those affected by an adverse event come together in a safe and supportive environment, with the help of skilled facilitators, to speak openly about what happened, to understand the human impacts, and to clarify responsibility for the actions required for healing and learning.'

Restorative approaches put patients and families at the centre of responding by asking all those involved what their needs are and establishing who is responsible for meeting them (Figure 4.3). Crucially, the process also recognises the importance of repairing the harm; not just the *physical harm* but also the *psychological or emotional harms* that can result from an incident. Finally, the process also asks those involved what might be done to prevent it happening again. In short, this approach centres the human needs of those affected by safety incidents, before coming to the question of learning and prevention.

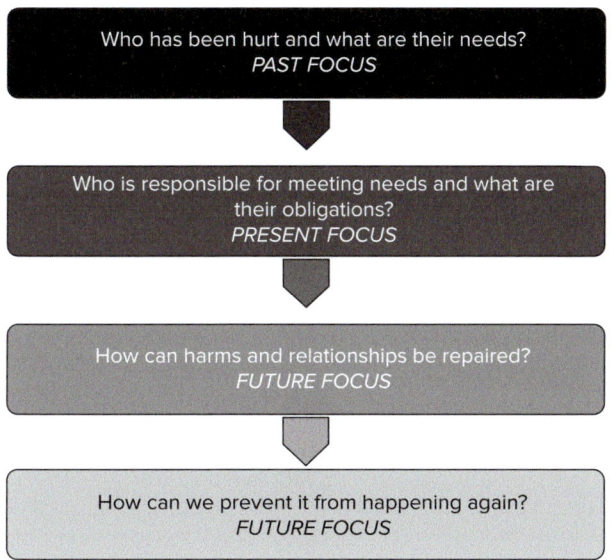

**Figure 4.3**   Restorative Enquiry Framework. (Wailling *et al.*, 2022; reproduced with permission.)

Whilst this type of approach is gaining increased interest, the evidence for its use — particularly at scale — is limited. It has been used successfully within a restorative response to surgical mesh harm in New Zealand (Wailling *et al.*, 2019; Wailling *et al.*, 2022). Following this, in 2023 a framework developed by the National Collaborative for Restorative Initiatives in Health was published to support the health and disability sector to mitigate and respond to healthcare harm in Aotearoa New Zealand. This is the first national health service to have embedded restorative principles (HQSC, 2023).

## Final Thoughts

Whilst healthcare is arguably different, and in some ways more complex than some of these sectors, it is clear that healthcare services can learn from the explicit, rights-based approach evident within such sectors. Having an explicit set of rights may well help focus attention and resources on involvement and engagement activity and affirm that those affected by incidents can have certain expectations following a patient safety incident. There are also important innovations emerging that have shaped, and will continue to do so, the future of involvement and engagement in incident responses within healthcare, both nationally and internationally.

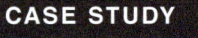

**CASE STUDY 1** — Patient Safety Manager from an Acute Trust

### Background

Traditionally in our Trust, involving families in an investigation following an incident — whether that's a 'minor' harm event or a 'serious incident' — has been limited. The family/patient may be 'allowed' to ask questions; however, they would not be directly involved in how the investigation was/is carried out.

These investigations are carried out by a team of clinicians/experts — we have 45 working days to complete a report. Once it has been signed off internally, via various committees, it will then be presented to the Integrated Care Board (ICB) for review within 60 days. The ICB will then close the report or ask further questions.

If the ICB and the Trust agree that the report can be closed, the report can then be shared with the family/patient. This sharing of the report constitutes the third stage of the Duty of Candour process.

Often, this will be the first time that the family/patient has seen this report. They are invited to discuss the report with the lead investigator.

These family meetings can be tense. The report can be a surprise for the family and may not even address the family/patient concerns. Some of the families'/patients' questions may not have been answered and the family view of events is not often considered. Further questions will arise as new information is presented to the family. This often leads to anger from the family, which may turn into a legal claim.

Part of the role of the patient safety manager at this Trust is to guide investigators through the process of completing the report and scheduling for various sign-off committees. These processes are determined by the Serious Incident Framework (SIF) set out by NHS England.

Traditionally, we have not involved the family or patient within the process of investigation as much as we could. Much of this may stem from beliefs that the Trust must protect its reputation and staff involved. If rigid processes that external and internal moderators impose are followed, this protects the Trust but is not conducive to a good relationship with the harmed patient/family.

The Duty of Candour process is mandated throughout the NHS in the UK. Every health and care professional must be open and honest with patients and people in their care when something goes wrong with their treatment or where care causes, or has the potential to cause, harm or distress. This means that health and care professionals must:

- tell the person (or, where appropriate, their advocate, carer or family) when something has gone wrong.
- apologise to the person (or, where appropriate, their advocate, carer or family).
- offer an appropriate remedy or support to put matters right (if possible).
- explain fully to the person (or, where appropriate, their advocate, carer or family) the short and long-term effects of what has happened.

These touch points with the family are usually the minimum that the family will receive; however, experience has shown this is not acceptable for either the family or the Trust.

As we implement PSIRF it has given us the perfect opportunity to try something different. Compassionate engagement is part of the PSIRF underpinning principles — in our Trust, we decided this was the time to do something different when involving families in incident investigation.

## What We Did

Our Trust had been considering the role of the FLO for a number of months. However, we did not know which model we would take — the mediation approach where the FLO would act as a mediator or the FLO as the investigator and the mediator?

Currently, the SIF is not set up for true family engagement. Governance processes in NHS Trusts are often rigid and have strict timeframes to follow. Families are not often ready to engage when we are, for many reasons, including the grieving process, family events or it's just not the right time.

As a team, including our director, we chose the FLO as a mediator approach. One of the patient safety team would be the family's one point of contact. It was assumed that the family would contact the FLO at any time during the investigation to ask questions, receive updates and review any draft reports; thus 'including' them in the process.

When contacting the family for the first time, the initial Duty of Candour was undertaken by the clinician involved. The family was then contacted by the FLO a few days later. We explained to the family that they could be involved in the investigation at every stage. The family were pleased, and we arranged a meeting with the investigating team.

The initial meeting did not go as well as expected. The family had already felt that the investigation had started without them. They were unaware of all the information. They felt that the Trust had all the information at their fingertips, whereas they were given information already screened by the Trust. They already felt an imbalance of power and became angry.

In turn, as the family became more frustrated, the more defensive the investigating team became — thus, increasing the anger of the family. Relations between the family and the investigation team was poor. All correspondence was through the FLO.

The FLO (mediator) was the 'middle man' who was trying to act as a 'bridge' between the investigating team and the family, rather than building a relationship which was equal, compassionate and engaging.

The family were unsure of what involvement actually meant. They were under the impression that the terms of reference would be set out with them — that they would able to interview staff, they would have regular updates from the investigator, they would be able to ask questions at any time, they would have access to the investigating team all the way through the investigation, they would have oversight on all drafts of the report and they would have an input on the actions.

Whereas the investigating team thought that family involvement meant answering the family's questions within the report and sharing back the final result. The investigating team were not available to the family; the investigating team were also clinical so were not solely working on the investigation. The investigating team became frustrated at the sporadic questions that were coming in from the family and were reluctant to share the draft report with the family until everyone was happy with it.

Meanwhile, the FLO was caught in the middle: trying to appease the family and the investigating team and seeing both perspectives, apologising to both parties at alternating instances.

## Lessons Learned

Usually, families would be contacted at the beginning of the investigation to ascertain any questions they had. They would then be given a copy of the report once it had been signed off by the Trust and the ICB. This process was often lengthy due to delays. The families were often kept at 'arm's length'.

By introducing the FLO we thought that the family would be involved in the investigation, there would be less delays and that the family would feel included; thus, aiding the healing process. However, trialling the role of a FLO as a mediator did not go as planned. In fact, it made the relationship between the family and the Trust worse.

The introduction of a FLO in this case resulted in unrealistic expectations from the family and the investigating team. Offering the family full involvement in the investigation but not giving any definition of what this actually meant to them, or the investigating team, set unrealistic expectations on both parties.

The investigating team were used to the old 'rules' and were reluctant to share any report with an outside source unless it had been signed off and had followed all governance processes. By not following these governance processes the investigating team felt exposed and vulnerable

### Tips:

- Consider the model of family liaison before any implementation.
- Set realistic expectations between the investigating team and family.
- Set out terms of reference together.
- Discuss with your executive team how you plan to involve families.
- Revisit governance processes around the sharing of reports and family engagement.

## Evaluation and Impact

This trial was carried out on a single case and we documented the feedback.

Feedback from the family:

- They had nothing to compare it to. They were grateful for the swift responses from the FLO; however, they did not feel involved in the investigation.
- They did not have the level of involvement that they expected.

Feedback from investigating team:

- They understand that the current processes are not set up for family involvement.
- They are keen to implement a FLO; however, they would like to agree governance processes with executive team.

Feedback from FLO:

- They felt like the 'middle man'.
- They did not feel that this model was the right one for this case.
- They felt like a glorified secretary at times.
- They did not feel they had any training to prepare them for this role.

## Conclusions

Following a patient safety incident, patients and their families require an apology, an understanding of what happened, meaningful involvement and compassionate engagement throughout the whole process.

An exploration of the appropriate model of family liaison used within the Trust where you work is vital for its success. The right training for this specialist role is also key.

We found there was a disconnect between what the safety team was intending to do and how the Trust expected the process to go. The safety team were trying to include the family at multiple points in the investigation; however, the Trust was hesitant to share any reports without the sign-off from all committees.

For patients and families to be involved with the investigation post-incident there needs to be reliance on outside influences and changing safety culture.

The experience of using this model of FLO for this one case was useful. We learned that this is a highly specialised role and one that required full support of the executive board. Understanding boundaries and managing expectations is key to success.

In the future, we will be advertising for two FLOs to work alongside complaints, patient safety and inquests. This joined up approach will aid the family to navigate through the complex systems and processes.

## Reflections from the Frontline

- Patient and family involvement in incident investigation is an essential part of PSIRF and the wider Patient Safety strategy. There are several models of involvement identified and good examples of engaging with families from outside the NHS and outside the UK.
- There are two main challenges to engaging patients and families: the level of involvement they want in an investigation and the level of training staff have. As outlined in the case study, if staff do not have adequate training, then it is incredibly difficult to engage appropriately. Each situation is unique, and each case may require a different level of involvement. The key is staff being able to successfully identify the needs of those they're involving and continue the engagement throughout the investigation process.
- There is no one way or model to engage and involve families. For example, a patient safety incident in a maternity ward will be different to an incident in a mental health setting, and it is important to understand how different settings might create different needs and expectations. Understanding these differences can help organisations know how to undertake involvement and engagement in ways that are inclusive and appropriate.
- Without adequate training, engagement with patients and families is incredibly challenging. Even with experience of engaging with patients and families in a frontline role, it may not adequately prepare someone for the level of post-incident connection that is required to successfully work together during an investigation. Initiatives like the Learn Together Programme are vital but will require adequate time and resource spent by Trusts to ensure the best practice is embedded in investigation teams and developed based on the client groups frequently involved. More specific guidance to support implementation would be valuable.

Funding statement: The Learn Together project is funded by the National Institute for Health and Care Research (NIHR) Health Services Delivery Research programme [18/10/02]. Lauren Ramsey and Jane O'Hara are supported by NIHR Yorkshire and Humber Patient Safety Research Collaboration (PSRC). The views expressed are those of the author(s) and not necessarily those of the NIHR or the Department of Health and Social Care.

## References

Bell, S.K. *et al.* (2012). 'Disclosure, apology, and offer programs: stakeholders' views of barriers to and strategies for broad implementation' in *The Milbank Quarterly*, 90(4), pp. 682–705.

Bismark, M. and Paterson, R. (2005). '"Doing the right thing" after an adverse event' in *The New Zealand Medical Journal* (Online), 118(1219):U1593.

Bismark, M. and Dauer, E.A. (2006). 'Motivations for medico-legal action: lessons from New Zealand' in *The Journal of Legal Medicine*, 27(1), pp. 55–70.

Etchegaray, J.M. et al. (2016). 'Patients as partners in learning from unexpected events' in *Health Services Research*, 51, pp. 2600–2614.

Harrison R., Birks, Y., Bosanquet, K. et al. (2017). 'Enacting open disclosure in the UK National Health Service: a qualitative exploration' in *Journal of Evaluation in Clinical Practice*, 23, pp. 713–718.

Health Quality & Safety Commission (2023). *He maungarongo ki ngā iwi. Envisioning a restorative health system in Aotearoa New Zealand*. https://www.hqsc.govt.nz/resources/resource-library/he-maungarongo-ki-nga-iwi-envisioning-a-restorative-health-system-in-aotearoa-new-zealand/.

HSIB. (2020). *National Learning Report Giving families a voice: HSIB's approach to patient and family engagement during investigations*. Healthcare Safety Investigation Branch I2020/007. https://www.hssib.org.uk/patient-safety-investigations/giving-families-a-voice/investigation-report/.

Iedema, R. et al. (2008). 'Patients' and family members' experiences of open disclosure following adverse events' in *International Journal for Quality Health Care*, 20: pp. 421–432.

Iedema, R. et al. (2012). 'What do patients and relatives know about problems and failures in care?' in *BMJ Quality & Safety*, 21(3), pp. 198–205.

Kok, J., Leistikow, I. and Bal, R. (2018). 'Patient and family engagement in incident investigations: exploring hospital manager and incident investigators' experiences and challenges' in *Journal of Health Services Research & Policy*, 23(4), pp. 252–261.

Louch, G. et al. (2021). 'Exploring patient safety outcomes for people with learning disabilities in acute hospital settings: a scoping review' in *BMJ Open*, 11(5), e047102.

McQueen, J.M. et al. (2022). 'Adverse event reviews in healthcare: what matters to patients and their family? A qualitative study exploring the perspective of patients and family' in *BMJ Open*, 12(5), e060158.

Mello, M.M. et al. (2014). 'Implementing hospital-based communication-and-resolution programs: lessons learned in New York City' in *Health Affairs* 33: pp. 30–38.

Mello, M.M. et al. (2016). 'Challenges of implementing a communication-and-resolution program where multiple organizations must cooperate' in *Health Services Research*, 51, pp. 2550–2568.

Mello, M.M. et al. (2020). 'Ensuring successful implementation of communication-and-resolution programmes' in *BMJ Quality & Safety*, 29(11), pp. 895–904.

Moore, J. and Mello, M.M. (2017). 'Improving reconciliation following medical injury: a qualitative study of responses to patient safety incidents in New Zealand' in *BMJ Quality & Safety*, 26: pp. 788–798.

Ockenden, D. (2020). *Emerging findings and recommendations from the independent review of maternity services at the Shrewsbury and Telford Hospital NHS Trust*. www.donnaockenden.com/downloads/news/2020/12/ockenden-report.pdf.

O'Hara, J.K. et al. (2018). 'What can patients tell us about the quality and safety of hospital care? Findings from a UK multicentre survey study' in *BMJ Quality & Safety*, 27(9), pp. 673–682.

Ottosen, M.J. et al. (2016). 'Developing the improving post-event analysis and communication together (IMPACT) tool to involve patients and families in post-event analysis' in *Journal of Nursing & Interprofessional Leadership in Quality & Safety*, 1:5.

Parliamentary and Health Service Ombudsman (PHSO). (2023). *Broken trust: making patient safety more than just a promise*. London, UK: Parliamentary and Health Service Ombudsman (PHSO).

Ramsey, L. et al. (2022a). 'Patient and family involvement in serious incident investigations from the perspectives of key stakeholders: a review of the qualitative evidence' in *Journal of Patient Safety*, 18(8), e1203.

Ramsey, L. et al. (2022b). 'Systemic safety inequities for people with learning disabilities: a qualitative integrative analysis of the experiences of English health and social care for people with learning disabilities, their families and carers' in *International Journal for Equity in Health*, 21(1), pp. 1–12.

Scottish Public Service Obudsman. (no date). *Meaningful apologies*. www.spso.org.uk/meaningful-apologies.

Vincent, C. et al. (2017). 'Safety analysis over time: seven major changes to adverse event investigation' in *Implementation Science*, 12, pp. 1–10.

Wailling, J., Marshall, C. and Wilkinson, J. (2019). *Hearing and responding to the stories of survivors of surgical mesh: Ngā kōrero a ngā mōrehu – he urupare*. (A report for the Ministry of Health.) Wellington, New Zealand: The Diana Unwin Chair in Restorative Justice, Victoria University of Wellington.

Wailling, J. *et al.* (2022). 'Humanizing harm: Using a restorative approach to heal and learn from adverse events' in *Health Expectations*, 25(4), pp. 1192–1199.

Weingart, S.N. *et al.* (2005). 'What can hospitalized patients tell us about adverse events? Learning from patient-reported incidents' in *Journal of General Internal Medicine*, 20(9), pp. 830–836.

Weissman, J.S. *et al.* (2008). 'Comparing patient-reported hospital adverse events with medical record review: do patients know something that hospitals do not?' in *Annals of Internal Medicine*, 149(2), pp. 100–108.

Wiig, S., Hibbert P., Braithwaite, J. (2020). 'The patient died: What about involvement in the investigation process?' in *International Journal for Quality in Health Care*, 17;32(5), pp. 342–346.

Wiig, S. *et al.* (2021a). 'Next of kin involvement in regulatory investigation of adverse events that caused patient death: A process evaluation (Part I – The next of kin's perspective) ' in *Journal of Patient Safety*, 17(8): e1713–e1718.

Wiig, S. *et al.* (2021b). 'Next of kin involvement in regulatory investigation of adverse events that caused patient death: A process evaluation (Part II – the inspectors' perspective)' in *Journal of Patient Safety*, 17(8), pp. e1707–e1712.

# CHAPTER 5

# Safety-II

*Mark Sujan*

## Summary

Safety-II has become a much talked about term in patient safety and healthcare quality improvement. Why certain concepts spark greater interest than others is often not entirely clear, but there is hardly a patient safety meeting or course where Safety-II is not at least mentioned. People are talking about adopting Safety-II, implementing or doing Safety-II, sometimes in a casual way like one would talk about, say, a new diet or fitness regime. However, Safety-II is not a method or an intervention, but rather a way of thinking about safety, a different perspective that can potentially provide novel insights about how complex systems work and about how they mostly succeed and sometimes fail.

This chapter will summarise the background to Safety-II and what 'doing' Safety-II might look like in practice. It will also discuss some of the potential pitfalls and issues that are yet unresolved, keeping in mind that the practical experiences of applying Safety-II in healthcare are still relatively limited. However, before we can talk about Safety-II, we need to have a brief look at Safety-I.

## Background

### There is No Safety-I

The term Safety-II seems to imply that, surely, there must be Safety-I. However, there is no Safety-I. What we have is a rich diversity of concepts, models and methods within safety science, which have been developed over the past 100 years (Dekker, 2019). It would be overly reductionist and counterproductive to label all these approaches simply as 'Safety-I' and move on to Safety-II as a new approach.

However, what we can observe is that certainly the early concepts and models, such as Heinrich's Domino model (developed in the 1930s), and also, to a certain extent, later models, including Reason's Organisational Accident model and Swiss Cheese model (developed during the 1980s and 1990s), adopted a definition of safety, which can be broadly summarised as the absence of accidents (Reason, 1997). An organisation is safe when it has minimised the number and severity of accidents.

From this perspective, negative outcomes, i.e. accidents, are the starting point for safety management. That is not to suggest that these approaches are purely reactive. The opposite is true. Approaches rooted in Safety-I thinking are very much proactive. However, the accident (real or hypothetical) is the focal point. We might start with the (hypothetical) accident and reason backwards about potential causes, or we might start with potential failures and reason forward to consider the impact of failures and how they might lead to accidents.

As the future is uncertain (i.e. we do not know if and when there will be an accident), the safety management principle is based on the concept of risk. Risk science is its own active scientific domain, and the depth of debate on risk is beyond what we need to consider for this chapter (for example, see Aven (2012) for further detail). Simplifying, risk is often operationalised in terms of the likelihood of occurrence of an event (e.g. a failure) and the severity of the associated consequences. Risk matrices are an example of this.

Safety management based on Safety-I thinking (i.e. centred on accidents and associated risk), is, therefore, concerned with the identification, evaluation and control of risk in order to reduce risk to acceptable levels. In UK safety-critical industries, acceptability of risk is usually defined through the so-called ALARP 'as low as reasonably practicable' principle (Sujan et al., 2016b). In essence, this means that (i) there are no intolerable risks in a system and (ii) other risks have been reduced to levels where further risk reduction would incur costs that are grossly disproportionate to the benefits.

So, despite the diversity and heterogeneity of approaches in safety science, when we say 'Safety-I', we refer to some basic high-level similarities these approaches share in terms of how they define safety and operationalise safety management. These are the focus on accidents and failures, and the control of risk.

## Why Do We Need Safety-II?

Looking at the history of safety science, there is a theme that runs alongside the development of concepts and models: complexity. The early approaches tended to represent and model organisations and accidents (i.e. lack of safety) in a relatively reductionist and deterministic way. They make use of models of systems based on the assumption that a system can be decomposed into its constituent parts and that these can be analysed in isolation.

In practice, this means that the system models we work with are often idealised and decontextualised representations of how we believe a system works, or, in other words, 'work as imagined' (Hollnagel, 2015). 'Work as imagined' describes the functioning of a system in terms of the rules and procedures that are in place, and which govern how work is supposed to be carried out. Based on this idealised and highly simplified description of the system, it is then attempted to identify potential vulnerabilities and failures in individual task steps or in specific components (e.g. equipment failures).

However, what people have realised over the years is that modern systems are more complex than can be represented in this reductionist way. As there is so much uncertainty in the environment of a system, the system design and the rules and procedures (i.e. work as imagined) are not perfect descriptions of how the system functions. Neither can outcomes be understood by simply looking at the functioning of individual system elements in isolation.

The increasing recognition of system complexity has been incorporated into safety science approaches since around the 1970s; that is, in thinking pre-dating Safety-II. Safety-II can be seen as one evolution of this thinking (there are others). Scholars including Jens Rasmussen, David Woods and Erik Hollnagel highlighted the importance of considering the interactions between different elements of the system. Rasmussen framed risk management in modern systems as a control problem, where the system is subject to a range of forces such as financial pressures, workload and capacity limitations, and safety concerns (Rasmussen, 1997). Hollnagel and Woods coined the term 'joint cognitive systems', emphasising the tight coupling between people, tasks, and the tools and technology people use (Hollnagel and Woods, 1983). To a certain extent, joint cognitive systems can be regarded as an earlier expression of what is now captured elegantly in the SEIPS model (Carayon et al., 2006) as elements of the work system and their interactions, but the thinking dates back over 40 years ago.

Hence, in some way, Safety-II is needed because systems are complex and full of uncertainty. In this respect, Safety-II can be regarded simply as an extension of thinking that started to be developed in the 1970s and 1980s. However, in other ways, there is a bit more to Safety-II than that.

## What is Safety-II?

At the start of this millennium, several researchers and safety practitioners came together in a workshop to debate the future of safety management in increasingly complex systems. Despite differences in their backgrounds, they shared the concern that existing approaches were inadequate to manage risk in such complex systems. This is because complex systems can fail in ways not represented in earlier models; for example, through dysfunctional interactions where no individual component might have failed, but the system still has an accident. From this, a new concept and a new discipline within safety science were created: resilience and resilience engineering (Hollnagel et al., 2006).

The term resilience has been used in different disciplines before and in different ways. In terms of resilience engineering, resilience refers to the ability of a system to 'recognise, adapt and absorb variations, changes, disturbances and surprises' (Woods and Hollnagel, 2006). This characterisation of resilience was then developed further by Hollnagel as the four cornerstones of resilience engineering (Hollnagel, 2010), or the four resilience abilities: the ability to anticipate, to adapt, to monitor and to learn.

Even within the community of resilience engineering, differences in perspective exist, and scholars went on to emphasise and develop different aspects. For Leveson, Rasmussen's concept of safety as a control problem remained central. This is reflected in Leveson's STAMP model (Systems-Theoretic Accident Model and Processes), which describes safety in terms of constraints which need to be actively maintained, and system behaviour controlled accordingly (Leveson, 2012). In this perspective, accidents happen when safety constraints are violated.

However, Hollnagel focused on developing the concept of safety not as the absence of accidents, but rather as the presence of resilience abilities. Hollnagel argues that it is impossible to study the absence of something (e.g. accidents and adverse events); instead we need to focus on that which is present. Hence, safety should be defined as the presence of something, and in this interpretation it is the presence of the ability to anticipate, to adapt, to monitor and to learn, or — in other words — the ability to succeed under varying conditions (Hollnagel, 2014). This definition of safety as the presence of abilities rather than the absence of accidents characterises the distinction between Safety-I and Safety-II.

From the definition of safety as the presence of abilities rather than the absence of accidents or unacceptable levels of risk, follows a different approach to how one manages safety. Rather than focusing on identifying, evaluating and controlling risk through engineered barriers and safeguards, and protocols and procedures aimed at standardising and constraining human performance, safety management under a Safety-II perspective is concerned with understanding performance variability and creating conditions that foster the ability to succeed.

The concept of performance variability is crucial to safety management within Safety-II. Owing to the complexity of modern systems and their need for flexibility and adaptability, it is impossible to design and describe in detail a system capable of managing all potential situations. Rather, people in the system are creating success in their everyday work through dynamic trade-offs and adaptations as they are managing competing organisational priorities and other mismatches; for example, in demand and capacity (Sujan et al., 2015). Usually, this performance variability is unremarkable and often invisible. However, on occasion, small everyday performance variability can reinforce itself to the extent that it becomes visible in the form of an incident or accident (Hollnagel, 2012). This is a non-linear property of complex systems in as far as otherwise undetectable weak signals (i.e. everyday performance variability) can lead to strong and undesirable system behaviours (i.e. accidents). Therefore, the view within Safety-II is that performance variability is both inevitable and generally useful, and that it is the source of both success and failure.

## Applying Safety-II

What, then, does 'doing' Safety-II look like in practice and what pitfalls are there? First of all, a word of caution — as these are relatively new concepts in patient safety (even if the roots date back decades), the practical experiences and the evidence base remain fragmented and weak (Verhagen *et al.*, 2022). However, this should not discourage practitioners from applying Safety-II to their own practice and to contribute their experiences to the debate.

### Understanding 'Work As Done'

Safety-II thinking assumes that 'work as done' by practitioners is necessarily different from 'work as imagined' as expressed in procedures and protocols. As described above, this is because of the complexity of systems and the inherent uncertainty. In practice, people have to make trade-offs, adapt to changing conditions and manage potentially competing priorities and goals.

From a Safety-II perspective, understanding work as done and appreciating the gap that exists between work as imagined and work as done is central. That is not to say that the gap can be eliminated. However, reflection on the work as imagined and work as done gap can help stakeholders from different backgrounds and with different perspectives develop a shared understanding of their collaborative work.

The Functional Resonance Analysis Method (FRAM) (Hollnagel, 2012) is a method that is increasingly being used in healthcare settings to study work as done (Sujan *et al.*, 2023). FRAM puts emphasis on exploring how work is carried out in practice, along with the normal variability resulting from trade-offs and adaptations, and the numerous functional interactions within a system. A FRAM analysis typically involves: (i) identification of functions; (ii) description of performance variability of each function; (iii) analysis of couplings between functions; and (iv) development of interventions to increase resilience. It is worth contrasting the focus on performance variability in FRAM with the traditional focus (i.e. in Safety-I thinking) on errors and failures.

For example, Schutijser and colleagues (Schutijser *et al.*, 2019) used FRAM to contrast work as imagined and work as done of the double-checking process involved in injectable medication administration. They collected data about work as imagined from protocols, and data about work as done through observations and group interviews. The 'work as done' model identified additional functions and was helpful to illustrate trade-offs in everyday work, which explain observed performance variability. They suggest that this was useful to practitioners as a starting point for developing improvement interventions.

### Learning from Everyday Work

A second example of how one can implement Safety-II thinking in practice is around organisational learning and incident response (Sujan *et al.*, 2017). Healthcare providers typically attempt to learn from retrospective analysis of incidents and adverse events through incident reporting systems and investigations based on approaches such as RCA. However, there is now a wealth of evidence available that healthcare providers are struggling to generate actionable learning from these activities and that they fail to implement sustainable improvements in practice (Sujan, 2015). There are many reasons for this, including a persistent blame culture and interventions that are targeted at the individual (e.g. further training and additional procedures) rather than at the wider system (Kellogg *et al.*, 2017).

From a Safety-II perspective, the focus on incidents and adverse events, (i.e. on negative outcomes), is misguided (Sujan, 2018). At best, these events can act as the starting point for further investigation, but the learning that can be derived from looking at negative events alone will always be limited. Instead, we should consider what ordinary, uneventful work looks like, because only the analysis of work as done on an everyday basis allows a deeper understanding of how a system normally functions and why it usually succeeds. Often, such an analysis of work as done can provide rich descriptive accounts of the adaptive strategies that healthcare workers adopt, such as sacrificing and reformulating goals, offloading of demands, pulling in extra resources, and trading off risks based on subjective assessments of the needs of a clinical situation (Sujan, 2022; Sujan et al., 2016a).

For example, during the early stages of the Covid-19 pandemic, the Chartered Institute of Ergonomics and Human Factors (CIEHF) developed guidance for organisational learning based on Safety-II thinking (Sujan et al., 2020, Sujan et al., 2021), which is highly compatible with the approach promoted within the new NHS PSIRF. Safety-II thinking appears ideally suited to capture, document and learn from the many adaptations that people made during Covid-19 (i.e. work as done), but the guidance is applicable to any context for organisational learning. The guidance frames organisational learning in terms of both the organisational mindset and the actions or the process to implement it (Figure 5.1). The mindset is about how an organisation approaches organisational learning. The guidance contains prompts to encourage organisations to think about their learning goals, who is involved in organisational learning, how deep their learning is, the types of situations they try to learn from and the

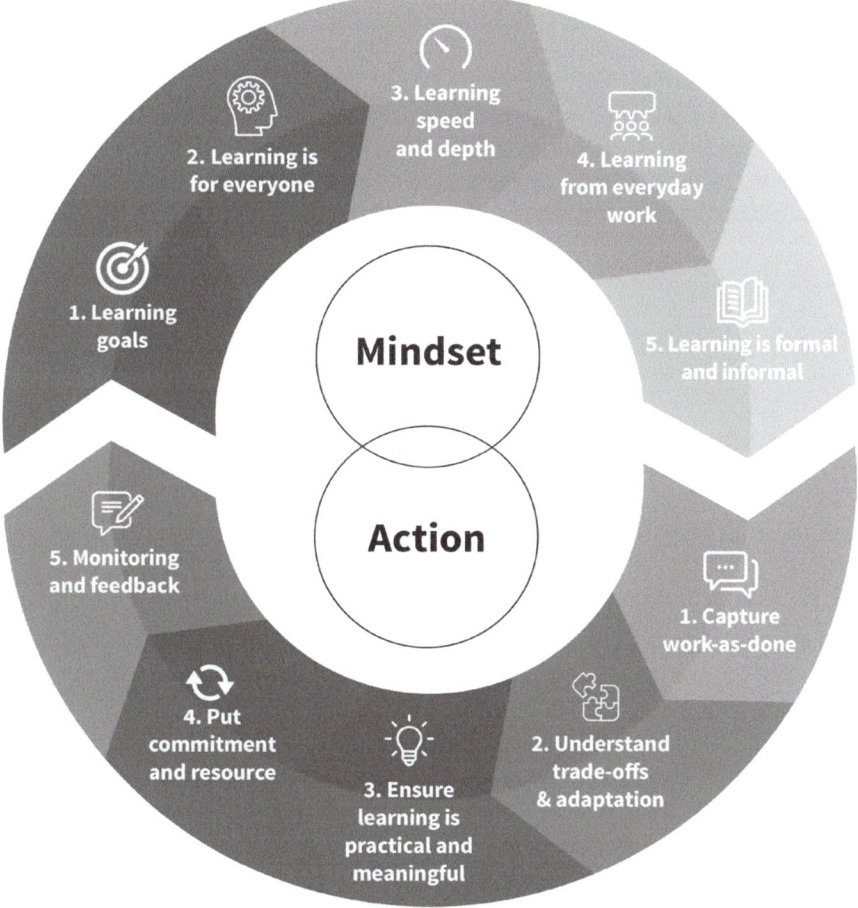

**Figure 5.1** The Chief Organisational Learning Framework for Achieving Sustainable Change, Achieving Sustainable Change: Capturing Lessons from COVID-19; 2020 © Chartered Institute of Ergonomics & Human Factors (CIEHF). Found online here: https://ergonomics.org.uk/asset/157D7305%2DD922%2D4215%2DB829BDD516FFB53D/

processes they have in place to foster learning. The actions describe how organisational learning actually takes place in an organisation, or how it is carried out. The guidance puts emphasis on learning from everyday work (rather than just from incidents) in order to understand how people adapt to situations and changes. It emphasises that staff should have an active role to play in organisational learning in order to ensure that learning is meaningfully related to practice and that, where possible, staff should be encouraged to take ownership for taking changes forward, and should be given authority and resources to do so. Finally, any changes that are implemented will likely require further adjustments over time, and therefore the learning process should be continuous and feedback from staff should be sought and given.

## Challenges in the Application of Safety-II Thinking

Despite the recent interest in Safety-II, in practice there is the potential for misinterpretation of Safety-II principles, and there is a lack of guidance as well as a limited evidence base. Verhagen and colleagues discuss some of the problems with making Safety-II work in practice (Verhagen *et al.*, 2022).

A key challenge for practitioners is how to balance Safety-I and Safety-II thinking: does Safety-II replace Safety-I, or can they co-exist, and, if so, how? From a practical perspective, it seems reasonable to suggest that a diversity of perspectives is a good thing, and, hence, the differences in Safety-I and Safety-II should contribute to better safety management. Although there can be tensions, the synergies that can be achieved are, arguably, much greater. For instance, failure analysis based on Safety-I thinking might suggest the introduction of a risk control; for example, in the form of a checklist or procedure. A Safety-II driven analysis can provide insights into work as done and how best to design flexibility into the checklist or procedure to ensure that the assumptions underpinning its development are more grounded in the realities and complexities of everyday work.

A second challenge concerns the development of safety improvements. Much of the literature on Safety-II describes analyses of work as done. Although this is helpful and insightful, it is not immediately obvious how the description of work as done then leads to interventions that improve safety. There is a danger that well-intentioned studies of work as done then lead to interventions that are very much aligned to Safety-I thinking. For example, the study of performance variability in a process could, potentially, be used to develop interventions aimed at constraining performance variability through the use of checklists and procedures. Such interventions would be more indicative of a Safety-I mindset rather than Safety-II thinking.

Lastly, as already alluded to, the scientific evidence base for Safety-II is still growing and, at the present time, remains fragmented. However, it is yet largely undocumented how specifically Safety-II has contributed to improved safety outcomes.

## Example of the Application of Safety-II in the Management of Deterioration

The application of Safety-II can be shown in a project that aimed to improve the management of patients who are at risk of deterioration following emergency surgery (Sujan *et al.*, 2022). Prior research demonstrated that the rate of complications following surgery is roughly comparable across different organisations (around one in four patients), but that the rate of patient death following complications can be much lower (about half) in successful hospitals compared with lower-performing hospitals (Ghaferi *et al.*, 2009). This means that some hospitals are better at recognising when a patient deteriorates and at escalating their care accordingly.

The rate of mortality following a complication is an important quality indicator and has been given a specific name — failure to rescue (Silber *et al.*, 1992). Accordingly, much of the research has been focused on identifying factors that contribute to failure to rescue; that is, factors that lead to negative outcomes (Box 5.1). Another way of looking at this issue, grounded in Safety-II thinking, is to study how the management of deterioration usually succeeds.

> **BOX 5.1** Common Recommendations to Reduce Failure to Rescue (Safety-I Thinking)
>
> **Failure to** notice patient is unwell → increase staffing levels
> **Failure to** measure vital signs → education & training
> **Failure to** calculate NEWS → education & training, usability
> **Failure to** take adequate history → education & training, staffing
> **Failure to** check notes → electronic medical records, usability
> **Failure to** commence correct initial treatment → education
> **Failure to** inform senior doctor → communication and teamwork
> **Failure to** arrange definite management → clear escalation protocol

The project studied how deterioration is usually managed (work as done) in a surgical emergency unit in an NHS hospital. The analysis used FRAM as the data collection and data analysis method. Data were collected through semi-structured interviews and workshops with a broad range of individuals and roles involved in the process.

The full detail of the study is described elsewhere (Sujan *et al.*, 2022). Here, we would like to focus on how recommendations for interventions were developed to contrast these with previous recommendations. Variability, in this project, was regarded only as the starting point for the analysis to enable understanding of the underlying system dynamics. The study was never concerned with whether variability was desirable or unwanted, but instead linked observed behaviours back to resilience theory; that is, the ability to anticipate, to monitor, to respond and to learn. The recommendations for improvement derived in this way focus on strengthening resilience abilities. Examples of recommendations are shown in Table 5.1.

**Table 5.1** Safety-II Recommendations for Managing Patient Deterioration

| Resilience Ability | Suggestions for Strengthening Resilience |
|---|---|
| Monitoring | • Dynamic plans for patients.<br>• Machine learning to predict deterioration.<br>• Create and maintain roles with explicit responsibility for having awareness of patients and patient movements across the department.<br>• Implement easily accessible and visible IT solutions (e.g. electronic whiteboard) that communicate this awareness to all relevant members of staff. |
| Responding | • Dynamic plans for patients – early involvement and starting escalation before patient deteriorates.<br>• Include roles that are deployable flexibly (e.g. floating staff).<br>• Rehearse and formalise which roles and which areas can provide resources during peak demand.<br>• Collaborative decision making and sharing of tasks (nurse – junior doctor).<br>• Facilitate bonding and relationship building. |
| Anticipating | • Implement IT systems that collect and aggregate relevant data. |
| Learning | • Implement organisational learning processes that capture everyday work.<br>• Design resilient procedures and work processes that explicitly consider the need for trade-offs.<br>• Create opportunities for informal and interdepartmental learning. |

Contrasting the recommendations derived from Safety-II thinking with those that have been previously made in the literature, we can see that prior recommendations typically establish a particular failure mode (e.g. failure to calculate the trigger score) and suggest barriers to prevent that particular failure (e.g. training, usability of tools). Often, these barriers are targeted at the individual. The recommendations based on Safety-II thinking are aimed at strengthening resilience by focusing on the resilience abilities. They do not, typically, take the form of barriers or risk controls, but aim to enhance the flexibility and adaptability of the system.

## Final Thoughts

Safety-II is not well understood by healthcare staff. A common misunderstanding is that Safety-II is only learning from when things go well. While Safety-II does explore the things that go well, it also uncovers *why* and *how* things go well and the interdependencies that allow this to happen.

The maturity of the safety culture in the healthcare setting will be dependent on how successful you are in changing the way you look at safety. Traditionally Safety-I has been a rather neat way of 'managing' incidents. The executive leads would be alerted to a serious incident, an investigation report written and action plan completed. Many of the actions would be around re-training and ensuring compliance with policy. If applying a Safety-II mindset the compliance data collected may become obsolete.

Currently, in the NHS in England the Clinical Negligence Scheme for Trusts (CNST) handles all clinical negligence claims against member NHS bodies. Although membership of the scheme is voluntary, all NHS Trusts in England currently belong to the scheme and compliance data is required to keep us covered — it's a little like an insurance. For example:

> 'Trusts that do not meet all ten safety actions will not recover their contribution to the CNST maternity incentive fund but may be eligible for a small discretionary payment from the scheme to help them to make progress against any actions they have not achieved. Such a payment would be at a much lower level their original 10 per cent contribution.' (NHS Resolution, 2023)

Many of these safety requirements involve compliance with policy. This approach is very much in keeping with the ultra-safe (avoiding risk) approach to safety (Vincent and Amalberti, 2016) which is a far cry from a Safety-II mindset.

Working in an ultra-safe/risk averse environment has challenges around psychological safety. This is defined by a positive safety culture as one where the environment is collaboratively crafted, created and nurtured so that everybody (individual staff, teams, patients, service users, families and carers) can flourish to ensure brilliant, safe care by continuous learning and improvement of safety risks, supportive and psychologically safe teamwork, enabling and empowering speaking up by all (NHS England, 2022).

Depending on where Trusts are along their safety culture journey will be dependent on how psychologically safe staff and patients feel. Observing and understanding everyday work will be easier for some to analyse, interpret and act on.

## Acknowledgements

This work was funded in part by the National Institute for Health and Care Research (NIHR) [Programme Grant for Applied Research NIHR200868]. The views expressed are those of the authors and not necessarily those of the NIHR or the Department of Health and Social Care.

## CHAPTER 5 ■ Safety-II

### CASE STUDY 1
Patient Safety Manager, Acute Trust

## Background

Patients who attend our hospital with both physical and mental health problems may be exposed to a sub-optimal experience compared to those that attend with a physical health issue only.

There had been numerous incident reports of recurrent self-harm, aggressive behaviour and absconding involving mental health patients within our Trust, which led to delays in physical health interventions.

Traditionally, these incidents would be investigated as an isolated incident, often with the immediate staff within that area. In some areas, such as the emergency department (ED), there are high numbers of these incidents.

The cycle of similar incidents being reported, reports written and similar action plans produced had been happening for years. There were many reasons for this:

- Treating mental health in an acute setting is not ideal: 'the shortage of mental health beds is the problem; we have no control over that.'
- This is a challenging problem that needs time — we don't have the time.
- Incidents can be closed quickly with re-training as an action.
- This is part of normal work — this is not an incident (under-reporting in some areas).
- Training staff is the answer — this assumes that staff are not able to care for these patients due to a knowledge gap.
- The assumption that a standard operating procedure (SOP) will fix it.
- Trust executive teams want reassurance that 'something' has been done to mitigate this from happening again — assurance seeking and a Safety-I mindset.

It was clear from the number of incidents, complaints, recurrent harm and poor experience from service users that the way we had been approaching the 'solution' was not working. With the introduction of PSIRF, it gave us the opportunity to 'investigate' differently.

There are numerous tools in the NHS England PSIRF toolkit, one of which is the After Action Review (AAR) (discussed in Chapter 6). The safety team decided to undertake an AAR to understand some of the issues that may not be captured during a regular RCA. We used the SEIPS framework (discussed in Chapter 3) to make sense of the wider systems that may have contributed to the incidents.

One of the actions from the AAR was to map the current pathway of the mental health patient as they come in through ED and then through the hospital to discharge. This initially started off as a regular process mapping exercise; however, the theory of Safety-II was at the forefront of the safety teams' minds after a recent teaching session.

The Safety-II concept was difficult to understand. The safety team had a misconception that Safety-II was learning from excellence and what goes right.

By clarifying with the wider safety team who were involved in the community of practice (the Patient Safety Managers Network) on what Safety-II was, we could start to implement the project. Within the community of practice there are several academics who have a deep understanding of the theory of Safety-II. Having access to academics was instrumental in trialling this approach. They were able to offer advice, challenge and support us through the process. Without this guidance, the team would not be confident in using this methodology.

### What Did We Want to Achieve?

The aim of this approach was to look at what policy and procedures we have written down (work as imagined) and to compare it with the everyday work (work as done) to understand the discrepancies. Our main aim was to enable staff to give good care, at the right time, to the right patient in ever-changing scenarios with the full support of the Trust.

Understanding the everyday work that staff undertake to enable the patient to 'move' through the hospital swiftly and with good care had not been explored previously. In terms of mental health, patients could be looked after by three different organisations under one roof. Each organisation had different staff, used different policies and different SOPs. Navigating this is difficult for staff, even more so for patients as they are unaware of how either organisation should function or that they were being seen by three different organisations.

There were three outcomes I wanted to achieve:

1. A shared purpose/aim of the workshops/project.
2. To create a psychologically safe environment for these workshops.
3. To shift the Safety-I mindset into the Safety-II mindset.

There were three outcomes I wanted the group to achieve:

1. Too understand and explore 'work as done' rather than 'work as imagined'.
2. A seamless pathway for mental health patients to move through the hospital system.
3. To create flexibility in the pathway to allow staff to adapt their decision making — removing 'safety clutter'.

## What We Did

Following the cluster of incidents, we did an AAR and a meeting was initiated to discuss the pathway of mental health patients coming in and leaving the hospital. Table 5.2 shows the type of staff involved.

The purpose of this meeting was to:

- Introduce the attendees to the Safety-II mindset.
- Set out scope for the project.
- Map out a high-level patient journey through the hospital.
- Understand who our stakeholders were.
- Pick out themes for further discussion.

Following this first meeting, I held three further meetings: one each week on the themes that were discussed. These themes were deemed the biggest issues that staff had:

- Triage and risk assessment.
- Referral.
- Escalating the patient with deteriorating mental health.

Table 5.2 Staff Invited and Involved in the Meeting

| Type of Staff | Invited | Attended | Reason for Non-Attendance |
|---|---|---|---|
| Staff from the Acute Trust (ED and the wards) Band 7 and below | Yes | No | Clinical pressure |
| Matron and lead nurses from ED and wards | Yes | Partial | Clinical pressure |
| Representation of the senior leadership team for nursing | Yes | Yes | N/A |
| Patient representatives/service users | Yes – after first meeting | Yes | N/A |
| Psychiatric liaison service | Yes | Yes | N/A |
| Drug and alcohol team | Yes | Yes | N/A |
| Director of Mental health | Yes | Partial | Clinical pressure |
| Psychiatrist | Yes | Partial | Clinical pressure |
| Security | Yes | No | Unclear |
| Violence and aggression matron | Yes | No | Clinical pressure |
| Patient experience team | Yes | Partial | Initial meeting |

Staff were more than willing to engage and participate as this had been an ongoing issue and they understood that traditional approaches to tackle this were not working.

To engage a specific patient group, namely a mental health group, it was important to get the service user involved rather than a generic patient group. By tapping into the local mental health advisory group, I was able to present my project proposal. There was a great response, and I had a small working group of three patients/carers.

I found Safety-II difficult to understand. I had assumed that I knew what Safety-II was; it is not around learning from excellence, but understanding what every day work is, how that work may change in different circumstances and how our decision making may change. It was daunting trying to explain this methodology to the mixed group, with limited knowledge myself.

I decided that the language that I used needed to be accessible. The word Safety-II seems nebulous — it means nothing without a huge explanation. These meetings were only 2 hours long, so I did not have time to explain in full. I made a conscious decision not use the term Safety-II until later in the meetings. Instead, I explained the different types of 'work': work as imagined, work as prescribed, work as disclosed, work as analysed, work as observed, work as simulated, work as instructed, work as measured and work as judged.

After explaining this, I demonstrated visually by sticking to the walls of the meeting room printouts of all policies/procedures/guidance that each staff member was expected to use. Altogether there were over 50. Some contradicted each other, some made little sense to the user, and some were out of date.

I asked questions such as:

- What conditions make this task easier?
- What makes your job harder?
- What gets in the way of you doing this task quickly/safely?
- Are there any 'tricks' you use to get the job done?
- What does the policy say, compared to what we do? Why is there a difference? Does this happen all the time? If not, when?

## Lessons Learned

There were several obstacles I faced where I had to subsequently make compromises. These are summarised in Table 5.3.

**Table 5.3** Obstacles Encountered and Compromises Made

| Obstacle | Compromise |
| --- | --- |
| Not all staff were able to make all sessions due to clinical commitments. | Individual catch-ups with missing team members post-meeting. |
| Executive team unclear on Safety-II approach and tried to push back to traditional methods. | Nil compromise. Education in Safety-II and reassurance in methodology. |
| Lower band staff unable to attend due to clinical commitments. | Top heavy in high management attendance, which may have limited free conversation. |
| Not enough time/staffing/cost. | Four 2-hour meetings to map pathway due to time/cost. |

Having a group of service users involved in a project was new to me. By inviting the patient experience team along to advise on how I invited patients and the practical implications — for example, their expenses and the language I used — was incredibly helpful. Ensuring that the patient group felt safe, at ease and welcomed was key in gaining their true perspectives.

## Tips

Creating a safe space for staff and patients to speak candidly on their everyday experience and work is paramount. Staff may feel uncomfortable telling the group that they may not always follow the policy, that they don't understand the SOPs or that there is a secret WhatsApp group of contacts as the Trust system is out of date. The safer the staff and patients feel, the richer the information you will glean. The executive team need to understand this approach and lead by example and support a methodology such as Safety-II.

Some staff were not comfortable in this candid approach and acted, at times, defensively. This was understandable but difficult to manage as it often led the others in the room to become defensive too.

Seeking support and clarification from outside my Trust was beneficial. Reassurance that I was on the right track from academics and from peers gave me the confidence to try this. Without this support my confidence in the approach and my ability would jeopardise the project. I was lucky enough to have an academic who specialises in this approach in the room with me to support me.

Your executive team will no doubt be nervous around this approach. Anxieties around regulation and compliance may pose a risk for them. Encouraging or condoning staff 'not following guidance' could leave them exposed for not following current policy. Although the benefits of this approach can be understood — the risk to the executive team may be too much.

## Evaluation and Impact

This project is ongoing; therefore it is too early to understand the impact this has had on services yet.

Since the time of writing, the Trust executives have read the initial report and have expedited the recommissioning of mental health services.

To progress the recommendations that will lead to improvement, four working groups were initiated: commissioning, patient experience, data gathering and processes. Within these working groups a gap analysis derived from the change ideas were listed. The working group will tackle each one. These working groups will then report into the original mental health Safety-II project lead for oversight.

## Conclusions

Facilitation of these meetings was difficult. Usually in a teaching session or a meeting you would have an agenda or plan, set with timings and centred around structured conversations. For this project, the loose plan of what we needed to focus on, keeping a Safety-II mindset and managing conversations was exceptionally challenging.

Psychological safety is key — we still have a way to go. Tackling a system problem, you need stakeholders from inside and outside your Trust. Creating an environment that crosses boundaries — location/organisational/professional — is new to us. These relationships need nurturing and that takes time.

This was our first project that crossed these boundaries and although relationships have been made, we are at the start of this journey. As time goes on, trust will build and allow for a more open conversation around work as done opposed to work as imagined.

Surprisingly, the patient group has been the most influential group. They are expecting an outcome, they are asking the tricky questions, they are challenging the status quo. With support from the patient experience team, they have a significant voice in this project.

If I were to undertake this approach again I would:

- Find a 'sponsor' from the executive team.
- Have a facilitator, a note taker and an observer to support me.
- Use different methodologies, such as small group work for more structured conversations.
- Have a smaller project.

## Reflections from the Frontline

- Safety-I and Safety-II don't have to be mutually exclusive; they are two perspectives that can each bring their own types of insights. However, it can be challenging to get people to look at a safety issue from different perspectives. Safety-I may be seen as 'bad' and it may be misinterpreted that we should only be looking from a Safety-II perspective; whereas, in reality, we should be looking at safety from all perspectives to gain a deeper understanding.
- This is a 'new' safety science for healthcare, so experts in this field are scarce. Modelling this mindset practically will take time. Ongoing coaching from the Organisational Development team may be required; however, they are not exposed to Safety-II and may find this a challenge.
- Education in the methodology and mindset of Safety-II is a good start. However, Safety-II is a shift in mindset and one that won't be shifted after a few hours of education. Thinking differently about safety takes effort and time; it is an iterative process and one that may take some months.
- The case study described that many of the policies sometimes contradicted each other, and many were unrealistic to follow; however, much of the time patients received safe care despite this. Staff were able to 'flex' the way that they work to adapt for differing times of day, staffing levels, capacity and demand for the service. Often the policies that are written are rigid and do not accommodate for any resilience in the system.
- Creating a safe space for staff and patients to speak candidly on their everyday experience and work is key. Staff may feel uncomfortable telling the group that they may not always follow the policy. The safer the staff and patients feel, the richer the information you will glean.
- Your executive team may understandably be nervous around this new approach and there will be anxieties around regulation and compliance, and they will need reassurance. Finding a 'champion' within the executive team will be important.

## References

Aven, T. (2012). 'The risk concept — historical and recent development trends' in *Reliability Engineering & System Safety*, 99, pp. 33–44.

Carayon, P. *et al.* (2006). 'Work system design for patient safety: the SEIPS model' in *BMJ Quality & Safety*, 15, pp. i50–i58.

Dekker, S. (2019). *Foundations of safety science: A century of understanding accidents and disasters.* Oxfordshire: Routledge.

Ghaferi, A.A., Birkmeyer, J.D. and Dimick, J.B. (2009). 'Complications, Failure to Rescue, and Mortality With Major Inpatient Surgery in Medicare Patients' in *Annals of Surgery*, 250.

Hollnagel, E. (2010). 'Prologue: The Scope of Resilience Engineering' in: Hollnagel, E. *et al.* (eds.) *Resilience Engineering in Practice: A Guidebook.* Farnham: Ashgate Publishing.

Hollnagel, E. (2012). *FRAM, the functional resonance analysis method: modelling complex socio-technical systems.* Farnham: Ashgate Publishing.

Hollnagel, E. (2014). *Safety-I and Safety-II.* Farnham: Ashgate Publishing.

Hollnagel, E. (2015). 'Why is Work as imagined different from Work as done?' in Wears, R., Hollnagel, E. and Braithwaite, J. (eds.) *The Resilience of Everyday Clinical Work.* Farnham: Ashgate Publishing.

Hollnagel, E. and Woods, D.D. (1983). 'Cognitive Systems Engineering: New wine in new bottles' in *International Journal of Man-Machine Studies*, 18, pp. 583–600.

Hollnagel, E., Woods, D.D. and Leveson, N. (2006). *Resilience Engineering: Concepts and Precepts.* Aldershot: Ashgate Publishing.

Kellogg, K.M. et al. (2017). 'Our current approach to root cause analysis: is it contributing to our failure to improve patient safety?' in *BMJ Quality & Safety*, 26, pp. 381–387.

Leveson, N. (2012). *Engineering a safer world*. Cambridge, MA: MIT Press.

NHS Resolution (2023). *Maternity Incentive Scheme – year five*. https://resolution.nhs.uk/wp-content/uploads/2023/07/MISyear5-update-July-2023.pdf

NHS England (2022). *Safety culture: Learning from best practice*. https://www.england.nhs.uk/long-read/safety-culture-learning-from-best-practice/

Rasmussen, J. (1997). 'Risk management in a dynamic society: a modelling problem' in *Safety science*, 27, pp. 183–213.

Reason, J. (1997). *Managing the risks of Organizational Accidents*. Farnham, Ashgate Publishing.

Schutijser, B.C.F.M. et al. (2019). 'Double checking injectable medication administration: Does the protocol fit clinical practice?' in *Safety Science*, 118, pp. 853–860.

Silber, J.H. et al. (1992). 'Hospital and Patient Characteristics Associated with Death after Surgery: A Study of Adverse Occurrence and Failure to Rescue' in *Medical Care*, 30, pp. 615–629.

Sujan, M. (2015). 'An organisation without a memory: A qualitative study of hospital staff perceptions on reporting and organisational learning for patient safety' in *Reliability Engineering & System Safety*, 144, pp. 45–52.

Sujan, M. (2018). 'A Safety-II Perspective on Organisational Learning in Healthcare Organisations; Comment on "False Dawns and New Horizons in Patient Safety Research and Practice"' in *International Journal of Health Policy and Management*, 7, pp. 662–666.

Sujan, M. (2022). 'Learning from Everyday Work: Making Organisations Safer by Supporting Staff in Sharing Lessons About Their Everyday Trade-offs and Adaptations' in Nemeth, C.P. & Hollnagel, E. (eds.) *Advancing Resilient Performance*. Cham: Springer International Publishing.

Sujan, M. et al. (2020). *Achieving sustainable change: Capturing lessons from COVID-19*. Wooton Waven: Chartered Institute of Ergonomics and Human Factors.

Sujan, M. et al. (2021). 'The contribution of human factors and ergonomics to the design and delivery of safe future healthcare' in *Future Healthcare Journal*, 8, e574.

Sujan, M. et al. (2022). 'Failure to rescue following emergency surgery: A FRAM analysis of the management of the deteriorating patient' in *Applied Ergonomics*, 98, 103608.

Sujan, M. et al. (2023). 'Operationalising FRAM in Healthcare: A critical reflection on practice' in *Safety Science*, 158, 105994.

Sujan, M., Pozzi, S. and Valbonesi, C. (2016a). 'Reporting and Learning: From Extraordinary to Ordinary' in Braithwaite, J., Wears, R. and Hollnagel, E. (eds.) *Resilient Health Care III: Reconciling Work as imagined with Work as done*. Farnham: Ashgate Publishing.

Sujan, M., Spurgeon, P. and Cooke, M. (2015). 'The role of dynamic trade-offs in creating safety — A qualitative study of handover across care boundaries in emergency care' in *Reliability Engineering & System Safety*, 141, pp. 54–62.

Sujan, M.A. et al. (2016b). 'Should healthcare providers do safety cases? Lessons from a cross-industry review of safety case practices' in *Safety Science*, 84, pp. 181–189.

Sujan, M.A., Huang, H. and Braithwaite, J. (2017). 'Learning from Incidents in Health Care: Critique from a Safety-II Perspective' in *Safety Science*, 99, pp. 115–121.

Verhagen, M.J., De Vos, M.S., Sujan, M. and Hamming, J.F. (2022). 'The problem with making Safety-II work in healthcare' in *BMJ Quality & Safety*, 31, pp. 402–408.

Vincent, C. and Amalberti, R. (2016). *Safer Healthcare. Strategies for the Real World*. Cham: Springer.

Woods, D.D. and Hollnagel, E. (2006). 'Prologue: Resilience Engineering Concepts' in Hollnagel, E., Woods, D.D. and Leveson, N. (eds.) *Resilience Engineering: Concepts and Precepts*. Aldershot: Ashgate Publishing.

CHAPTER 6

# After Action Review

*Judy Walker*

## Summary

An After Action Review (AAR) in a healthcare setting is a structured review process, undertaken primarily in groups, which seeks to identify and reinvest learning for improvement. Typically facilitated by a neutral AAR Conductor and undertaken in a single session, usually lasting an hour, the discussion in an AAR is focused on four questions. These questions seek to ascertain what staff expected would happen, what actually happened, why was there a difference between expected and actual experiences, and what can be learned from the event. AARs create opportunities to improve personal, team and organisational effectiveness, to deliver safer, better patient care, and to improve service user and staff experience.

This approach to learning can be classified as a 'Team Based Quality Review', which is a generic term used by NHS Scotland for multi professional learning activities or as a structured group debriefing process (Kumar, 2023).

This chapter will discuss the origins of AAR, the theory and research behind it, and the five components of AAR. It explains with examples and case studies how it can be implemented into practice.

## Background

The AAR originated in the US military during the second world war (Morrison and Meliza, 1999), when Brigadier General S.L.A. Marshall developed an 'interview after combat' technique where he assembled battle participants after the fighting had ended and conducted group interviews. Marshall's task was to provide accurate records of the battles. He realised that accounts from those in charge could only provide one part of the story; he needed to be able to capture a richer picture of events from those directly involved.

The AAR appears again in response to the challenges encountered in the Vietnam War (Salter and Klein, 2007) in the late 1960s. The thousands of Americans troops stationed in Vietnam had to learn quickly from their engagements with the Viet Cong. The Generals realised that this knowledge was an asset that needed to be shared up the chain of command, so they adapted the baseball match debrief, to hold what became AARs at the end of each engagement or 'action'.

> 'The After Action Review has democratised the Army. It has installed a discipline of relentlessly questioning everything we do. Above all it had re-socialised many generations of officers to move away from a command-and-control style of leadership to one that takes advantage of distributed intelligence.'
>
> Brigadier General W. Scott Wallace (Pascale *et al.*, 2001)

Darling, *et al.* (2005) report that AAR as we know it today began its life at the US Army's National Training Centre (NTC) in the 1970s where the use of frequent AARs during realistic battles proved highly effective, and AARs became a well-established part of both Army culture and standard procedure in both training and operational environments. As generations of soldiers rotated through the NTC, the methodology evolved and AARs eventually moved into the business world when former military leaders joined the management teams of major US corporations in the early 1990s.

The AAR was introduced into the NHS in England in 2008 (Walker *et al.*, 2012). A physician, Professor Aidan Halligan, who had witnessed its effective use in a military field hospital in Camp Bastion in Afghanistan, recognised its potential to radically improve patient safety by increasing team-based, ward-based learning after adverse events. He won the support of the hospital board at University College London Hospitals NHS Foundation Trust to fund a training programme, which hundreds of clinical and managerial staff participated in over several years. Once the success of the approach was recognised, other hospitals began to use it and in 2022 NHS England included it as one of the recommended Learning Response Tools in PSIRF.

## The Theory Behind the Practice of AAR

The same principles that led to the development of AAR in military settings apply to healthcare settings; frontline clinical and operational staff are learning every day. When learning is identified and shared within an AAR, that knowledge then becomes an organisational asset to support continuous improvement. In a similar way to the military, hierarchy needs to be removed from the learning process and the voices of all those involved in an action included.

Further principles that aide our understanding of the approach are articulated in a meta-analysis of 46 research papers into the impact of AAR (Tannenbaum and Cerasoli, 2013). They used four elements to determine whether a research paper could be included in the meta-analysis. These illustrate what is meant by an AAR and indicate the mechanisms through which AAR contributes to improving patient safety.

1. **Active (versus passive) Self-Learning**
AARs are a form of emergent learning in which individuals are actively involved in self-discovery and build their own understanding of how to improve performance. The AAR process enables clinical and operational staff to be active participants in making sense of the situations they have experienced. This creates the conditions for more lasting change compared with receiving feedback or someone else's interpretation of causal factors. This active self-learning enables individual staff to make safer 'micro' as well as 'macro' decisions and better judgements in their everyday activities.

Active self-learning refers to Kolb's experiential learning theory (Kolb, 1984). According to Kolb 'learning is a process, in which knowledge is created through transformation of experience'. The AAR process is designed to facilitate and enhance the learning cycle to support this transformation of experience. During the AAR process participants first reflect on their own and others' experiences and use this lens to get greater insight and understanding on what this experience means. Throughout the AAR and afterwards, abstract conceptualisation happens as the learner forms new ideas or adjusts their thinking based on the experience and their reflection about it. Once the AAR is completed, active experimentation begins where the learner applies the new ideas to the world around them. This process can happen over a short or long period of time.

## 2. Developmental (versus administrative) Intent
The developmental, nonpunitive focus of an AAR fosters an environment that encourages listening, honest information exchange and perspective taking, and maximises the potential to learn from experience. Participants in an AAR are not being told what to do differently, they are instead developing the concepts themselves. This applies to all participants, whatever their status in the hierarchy. The developmental context for the AAR is set by both the AAR Conductor, who facilitates the process, and by the organisation in which AAR is being applied. Leaders must endorse and value the focus on individual learning; this is a more democratic approach rather than administrative box ticking.

## 3. Specific (versus general) Events
Reflecting on specific incidents allows for a deeper examination of actions at the individual, team and system level, including both human and process factors, and allows for the creation of highly relevant action plans from the learning that takes place. If a patient safety or operational event was lengthy or complex, then several AARs might be conducted for the same event, each with a different specific area for focus.

## 4. Multiple (versus single) Information Sources
Those directly involved in a patient safety event will try to make sense of their individual experience and derive their own explanations for what has happened, but they will have an incomplete picture. Hearing from others directly involved in the incident allows for a more diverse and complete account of what occurred. This leads to learning about the context of the event for the individuals concerned and creates the opportunity for understanding the connections between one's own actions and those of others, and the context in which all were working.

Sociocultural theory, as its name indicates, holds that learning is an essentially social activity with processes and outcomes that have cultural and historical dimensions.

This fourth element helps to reduce the cognitive biases of participants and supports effective decision making as a result of the AAR. In the highly emotive context of healthcare delivery, inductive reasoning leads us to allocate causation, often in the form of blame as a default because we are biased by our own limited view of the event. The AAR process helps participants to make sense of the system in which the event occurred, and so the conditions are created to develop less biased, blame-laden perspectives. As Daniel Kahneman (2012) says, 'alternative descriptions of the same reality evoke different emotions and different associations'. Multiple information sources in an AAR ensure we move away from the narrow focus of our own experience to the wider perspective of the group's experience.

The success of the AAR approach in bringing about impactful change can also be explained by Knowles' Adult learning theory (Knowles et al., 1984). To learn effectively, adults must be active participants in their learning; topics must be relevant to the adult's own context; the work moves from a problem towards the solution and adults are able to make choices to bring about improvement. The correct application of the AAR approach meets all these conditions.

It is vital to ensure the conditions are right for learning; as Edmondson (1999) explains, learning is inhibited when we face the potential for threat or embarrassment. Our cognitive capacity is curtailed when we feel the need to be vigilant. However, when we feel psychologically safe, we don't need to perform the mental risk calculations and assess our vulnerability whenever we want to speak honestly or ask a question so can think more broadly and creatively. This is why so much of the work of the AAR Conductor and the organisation using AAR is focused on creating and maintaining psychological safety using the tools described below.

# The Five Components of the AAR

## 1. The Four Questions

The four questions of the AAR are divided into two phases: the descriptive phase, where participants get to listen to the expectations and the lived reality; and the evaluation phase, where the group does a 'gap analysis' between the intended outcomes and the lived reality. This means exploring the barriers to and enablers of performance, articulation of the learning that has arisen and decision making about what comes next. The best results come when the AAR Conductor ensures each of the four questions is explored in some depth before moving on to the next. This is because when the same question is asked over and over again, the participants will share more information and a greater understanding will be achieved.

*What was expected?* AARs in NHS settings differ from the military context because all military encounters have a 'mission', which describes the specific task or duty assigned to an individual, weapon or unit, so their AARs are largely undertaken against the details described in the mission. While there will be a plan, policy or clinical guidance for many of the things that healthcare staff do, these are rarely as detailed and specific as a military mission. This means that the first question isn't 'What was the plan' but 'What were we expecting?' Expectations of what will happen or should happen are constantly running in the background of our consciousness and inform our behaviour and experience of the world. Some are explicit expectations: for example, a nurse admitting a patient will be expected to undertake a set of standard procedures. Many are implicit, and shaped by experience, culture and context. For example, expectations about who has decision-making responsibilities within a team may vary. Because such things are rarely articulated, the expectations question is a powerful one for revealing the assumptions that were operating in the background and helps the participants see for themselves the similarities and differences between them.

The AAR Conductor's role is not to know whether the expectations expressed are reasonable or inappropriate, excessive or modest. The aim is that the individuals express their expectations, plans or imagined outcomes based on what is normal for them as an individual and within their role in healthcare and the AAR needs to ensure these are expressed and understood by all participants. This doesn't mean that the AAR should not include a discussion about what is a reasonable expectation. Once the AAR moves into the second half where creativity and action planning is required, the expectation question can be returned to in a different format.

*What actually happened?* The second question of the AAR is 'What actually happened?' and this provides an opportunity to build the bigger picture of the event through the multiple perspectives of everyone in the AAR. The scope and the time allowed for the AAR will guide how much of what actually happened is shared, but details of what was actually happening for the individual and what they saw, felt and heard will enrich the picture for the other participants. In some ways it is the easiest of the four questions because humans are very used to speaking about what they have experienced. However, people need to feel psychologically safe to be able to share their experiences in front of others, especially where these people are more senior or more junior to themselves. The AAR Conductor will need to ensure that 'what actually happened' refers back to the answers given in response to the expectations questions and may make specific links to this material if needed.

*Why was there a difference?* Next, the AAR moves into the evaluative phase with the third question seeking to understand 'Why there was a difference between what was expected and what actually happened?' This phase of the AAR is essentially a gap analysis to explore what happened between 'work as imagined' and 'work as done' (Dekker, 2014). This exploration normally takes the form of two 'what' questions, rather than the why question itself, to ensure a balanced view can emerge. The first is 'What got in the way of the expectations being met?' and invites participants to identify barriers to achieving the expected or desired results. Neither the AAR Conductor nor the participants should be judging or weighting the contribution of these barriers at this stage. The aim is to generate as many ideas as possible about what contributed to not being able to achieve the desired results. These will fall into two broad categories: those which were outside of the participants' control, such as staff shortages or the patient's behaviour, and those that might be within the participants' control, like how they responded to staff shortages or dealt with the patient's behaviour. These categorisations will be important in the final phase of the AAR.

The second 'why' section question aims to get clarity on the elements that enabled participants to achieve what was expected or the actions and behaviours that enabled things to go better than expected. Asking 'What enabled you to achieve what you did?' and 'What would you want to be repeated/retained if you were in this situation again?' encourages participants to identify the components of behaviours or actions that supported success. Again, the AAR Conductor may prompt people to refer back to key elements of the action and ask what might have contributed to that outcome.

Framing questions in this 'why' section as 'what' questions enables the participants to identify factors within the SEIPS framework (Carayon *et al.*, 2006) as the focus is not on the person or root cause, but on the context in which the patient safety event occurred. Framing the outputs within SEIPS may be made explicit within the AAR itself or through the AAR reporting template used. However, more commonly it is an implicit part of the process rather than an explicit one, with the AAR approach aligning with the SEIPS philosophy of learning about the situational, organisational and cultural factors. See Chapter 3 on SEIPS for more information.

*What have we learned?* The final phase of the AAR moves into identifying the learning and developing the actions arising from the learning. The open question 'What have we learned?' will stimulate a synthesis and sense-making response and socialise the learning in the group of participants.

To benefit future patients and teams, there needs also to be follow on questions: 'Given what we've learned, what might (or will) we do differently to prevent this happening in the future?' 'Given what we've learned, what might (or will) we do the same or more of in the future?' The aim is to use this material to get individuals to describe specifically what changes they are taking responsibility for and shape them into specific actions at the individual as well as team and organisational level, with names attached as appropriate.

The emphasis of the actions should be on things that are within the participants' own control, that will be done by them, as well as about the things they want to influence, as this is how patient safety will improve.

## 2. Scoping the Specific Purpose of the AAR

Creating the conditions for others to learn during an AAR requires clarity on the scope and purpose of the AAR so that sufficient depth of learning is achieved within the time allocated. Many patient safety events will seem to need little scoping, such as one for a patient fall, but it may be that the richest area for learning is not the events that led to the patient's fall itself but the team's response to it. For example, an AAR to learn from a patient who had an undiagnosed hip fracture after a fall might have a different focus to one where a patient fell when escorted by her family.

To scope the AAR, the AAR Conductor will need to discuss the action to be reviewed with the 'AAR Sponsor' or whoever called for the AAR. On some occasions, the specific purpose may instead be defined by the participants at the start of the AAR. The aim is to determine the richest areas for learning, themes to be explored, the timescale to be focused on and any areas of sensitivity to be alert to.

It is very likely that this scoping conversation will reflect some of the AAR Sponsor's own biases, but it is necessary to have a guide for the context of the AAR and it will assist the AAR Conductor in shaping the expectations question and the learning questions to meet the specific purpose. Adjusting the expectations question to the specific context will ensure that participants speak more specifically than generally. For example, an AAR called to learn from the response to a cardiac arrest (CA) in the front hall of the hospital, with a specific purpose to look at the practicalities of responding to CAs in novel locations might start with:

'What do you expect to have happen when there is a CA in the front hall?'

If the purpose was to look at roles and responsibilities, the first question might be:

'What do you expect people with your role to be doing when responding to a CA in a location like the front hall?'

The fourth question about learning can also vary depending on the outcomes suggested by the AAR Sponsor. Is the outcome to be focused on individual, team or organisational learning or all three? For example, if the sponsor is keen that individuals take responsibility and get involved in bringing about change then the learning question will include, '*What will you do as a result of this learning?*' Whereas if the sponsor wants the team to work together to bring about change as a result of the learning, then you might include '*What are you learning that needs to be done differently in this team?*'

## 3. The AAR Conductor

This term was given to the facilitator of an AAR, to identify it as a specific role with a defined remit, undertaken by those who have participated in training to ensure it is done professionally. The role of the AAR Conductor is to create the conditions for others to learn and to do so using specific techniques, tools and processes as well as through their own behaviour. The remit is to continuously improve the delivery of safe, effective patient care through the learning that takes place in the AAR. The metaphor of the orchestral conductor is helpful in bringing clarity to the AAR Conductor role (Table 6.1).

**Table 6.1** The Role of the AAR Conductor Using the Metaphor of the Orchestral Conductor

| | | |
|---|---|---|
| Silence | The Conductor of an orchestra or a choir is silent yet enables others to produce a coordinated sound. | The AAR Conductor is largely quiet speaking only to set the scene, ask the questions and to summarise periodically. Participants in the AAR 'make the music'. |
| Score | The Conductor uses a score to guide the musicians' journey together and has a clear understanding of all the elements of this score. | The AAR Conductor has the ground rules and the four questions to guide the participants through the learning journey. |
| Sensing | The Conductor is always sensing and connected to what is going on in the orchestra and the sound they are creating, responding as needed to improve the quality of what is heard. | The AAR Conductor is always sensing and listening to what is being said and expressed nonverbally, responding to quieten the 'trombone section' and ensure the 'piccolos' are heard. |

The role of AAR Conductor requires no knowledge of the topics to be explored. In fact, the lack of specialist knowledge can be seen as an advantage as it enables the AAR Conductor to ask genuine questions and work without any preconceived knowledge of their own. Conductors do need to have, and develop through expert training and experience, confidence to lead others through the AAR process and ask the same questions of those more senior to them as well as more junior. Another role requirement is the curiosity to ask questions and rapidly pursue lines of enquiry as the opportunities for exploration arise.

Participants in an AAR need to be able to trust that the AAR Conductor will ensure that the experience is a psychologically safe one, where people do not feel they are at risk of being blamed. The Conductor needs to be able to build trust by briefing the participants at the outset and owning the process throughout.

## 4. AAR Ground Rules

One of the ways in which the AAR Conductor creates a psychologically safe and productive learning environment is by first articulating and then implementing a set of universal ground rules. Normally these are verbally set out at the start by the AAR Conductor, and then used to maintain safety throughout. The standard ground rules are described below. These may be shortened for teams that use AAR routinely, but they should not be omitted entirely as they serve as a reminder of the behaviours expected during the AAR and a signal of the AAR Conductor's authority.

1. To build a full picture of the action, we need to assemble all pieces of the puzzle so I will be inviting each person to contribute in turn.
2. We have a finish time of … and it is my job to keep us to that so I may have to ask you to be brief sometimes, or I may interrupt you when you are speaking.
3. To get the most out of our time together, I ask that you are fully present and switch off your phones and emails and focus on listening and learning.
4. Our purpose here is not to investigate the past but instead to learn as a group and make decisions about what happens in the future. Please come with a curious and open mind, ready to reflect and learn together.
5. I expect you to give your own first-person account of what you were expecting and what actually happened and describe these from your own perspective. Please be as open and honest as you feel comfortable being.
6. This is a confidential learning environment. I encourage you to share your learning coming out of the AAR, but I do not expect you to share the details of what is discussed. A summary of the lessons learned and the topics covered will be written but nothing reported will be attributable to an individual.
7. Central to every AAR is this concept that hierarchy is left outside. We are all learners here, whatever our rank in the organisation and there is no hierarchy in learning.
8. While there may have been issues that arose that did not go as expected, we are not here to allocate blame on someone else, or ourselves. Blame is about the past and learning is about the future. That is what we are here to do. Learn for the future benefit of all.
9. Are we able to work together with these ground rules?

Challenges in implementing these ground rules will occur frequently and the AAR Conductor will need to point out these infringements as soon as possible to ensure psychological safety is maintained.

## 5. Participants

All those participating will arrive at the AAR with some preconceived ideas and possibly with some emotional reactions to the event itself. It is the role of the AAR Conductor to understand this and to be a professional and supportive presence as the AAR begins.

Each of those invited to the AAR should have had first-hand experience of the action to be reviewed but on occasion it can be valuable to include others not directly involved but who will help bring about change as a result of the AAR.

The number of participants in an AAR depends on the event itself and the scope of the AAR. More complex topics involving more people who had 'hands on the patient' will require longer than simpler topics where less people were involved. The more people who participate in the AAR, the greater the number who will be able to benefit from first-hand learning. The wider the diversity of roles and departments who participate, the richer the learning will be. However, the size of the group will affect the quality of attention and engagement achieved. If the listening time for individuals is much longer than the contributing time, the effectiveness of the AAR will be reduced.

## Patients and Family Members as Participants in AARs

Including patients and family members in AARs has the potential to significantly increase the richness of the learning as well as giving the patient reassurance that learning and change is taking place. It's also a highly effective mechanism for enabling patients to contribute to improvements. To be effective, decisions have to be made about when it's appropriate to invite them to participate. Exclusions may include:

1. When the patient or family members' emotional response to the event means they are not yet ready to contribute in the context of learning.
2. When the staff involved have been significantly affected by the event.
3. When an individual's action or inaction is the main cause of the event.

When a decision to include patients is made, then appropriate consultation needs to take place so that patients and family members understand the process and the purpose and ensure they can opt in or out at any point. See Chapter 4 on involving families.

## AAR Research

There has been considerable research into the practice of debriefing; defining the outcomes and benefits as well as the components which contribute to success. Some of these focus on structured approaches such as the AAR as a means of improving team performance and as a mechanism for increasing safety in high reliability organisations settings such as healthcare.

A quantitative meta-analysis of 46 pieces of published and unpublished research on team and individual level debriefs and AARs (Tannenbaum and Cerasoli, 2013) found that on average, debriefs improve the effectiveness of team performance over a control group by between 20 and 25 per cent. The analysis revealed a greater impact on team performance was achieved when there was alignment in terms of the AARs' specific focus on team or individual learning and the potential impact of the quality of facilitation and using a structured approach.

Renshaw *et al.* (2020) report on the use of AARs to help reduce the numbers of patient falls in a large acute hospital setting. AARs were led by a trained AAR Conductor, with all staff directly involved in each event as well as patients and family members wherever possible. The paper suggests that between 2011 and 2019 this approach has led to 5108 fewer falls and a saving of £13.3 million.

A review of team debriefings in healthcare by Kolbe *et al.* (2021) explores the need to differentiate between 'debriefing-to-treat' and 'debriefing-to-learn'. The latter does not prevent post-traumatic stress disorder (PTSD) and other psychological repercussions of a traumatic event and may cause harm. Debriefings held with the intended outcome of learning will foster sense making but since it may require respectful persistence by facilitators to explore uncomfortable topics, it is contraindicated when participants are distressed.

A survey-based study (Crowe, 2017) in the fire service in North America demonstrated that AARs conducted directly after a fire can improve fire crews' safety awareness. Part 1 of the study saw 119 firefighters responding to a survey asking, 'What makes a good After Action Review?' and "What makes a bad After Action Review?' The results were used to create a series of statements of attendee behaviours in AARs which a further 311 firefighters rated from their own experience. The results identified that good AAR attendee behaviour is positively related to AAR meeting satisfaction and group safety norms and that these relationships are dependent upon the frequency with which AARs are called by the crew leaders.

## Implementation

### Quality Issues

AARs need to be led by people trained to do so, to manage blame, hierarchy and fear and ensure the environment is a psychologically safe and inclusive one. People's trust in the process relies on the behaviour and skill of the AAR Conductor. Without trust in their abilities, the quality of engagement and learning will be lower. Alongside this, there needs to be organisational trust in the AAR process. Switching to this more democratic form of learning, where the power for change and responsibility for improvement is devolved down the traditional hierarchical ladder, needs to be endorsed at every level of the organisation.

### Legal Issues

As well as leadership engagement and a sustained communications strategy to develop this trust, there needs to be clarity on the legal context for the use of AAR within a healthcare setting to remove the fear of litigation. AAR sits under the umbrella of 'group reflection', and the General Medical Council (GMC) and the Nursing and Midwifery Council (NMC) issued a statement which clarified their common expectations for health and care professionals to be reflective practitioners (GMC, 2019).

Any notes taken as part of an AAR could, potentially, be disclosed as part of any litigation or legal process undertaken against a healthcare provider. Minute taking should not be done because of the 'safe space' environment that is required to facilitate more open discussion. However, the AAR Conductor may create a report on the topics covered, learning achieved and what has been agreed to serve as a reminder and meet governance requirements, but nothing reported should be attributable to an individual. The fact that an AAR has taken place should not be seen as prejudicial to the litigation as it is a widespread practice within the NHS. The clinical professions (GMC and NMC) also have Codes of Conduct that promote the value of learning as a mitigation activity after an incident, and as a leadership activity within the team (NMC, 2015).

## Final Thoughts

Once you have trained and experienced AAR Conductors and widespread trust and appreciation of the process in an organisation, decisions will need to be made about how to get maximum value from the regular use of the approach. When numerous AARs are taking place, the lessons learned and actions arising will be bringing about change and improvement locally but what about the learning from all the AARs? How might maximum value be gained from the themes and trends emerging through the volume of AARs?

Digital platforms are emerging that will help organisations see the wider picture of AAR activity. However, the input side of such AAR reporting tools must not compromise the open-ended exploration that characterises the AAR by being heavily prescriptive. To get an overall picture, organisations should establish governance processes that ensure themes emerging in a clinical specialty are collated. Periodic reviews of AAR reports by an AAR review team could also do the work of synthesis and theme identification. Trends can also be looked for such as where AARs are being held and what professionals and roles are engaging in them.

When AAR gains traction in an organisation, the use of AAR for learning from significant events leads to more regular use of AARs. The approach starts to be used to learn from low harm events, positive outcomes and a wide range of topics and operational issues unrelated to patient safety, shaping a 'continuous improvement' mindset. It also leads to increased awareness about multiple expectations operating prior to actions and so encourages the use of Before Action Review to create alignment and situational awareness *before* the activity begins. At an individual and team level there will be many surprising, highly valuable innovations and adaptations of the principles of AAR and these need to be socialised for the benefit of all.

## CASE STUDY 1

Katy Fisher, Wrightington, Wigan and Leigh NHS Foundation Trust

### Background

Our Trust, in collaboration with a Mental Health Trust, had trialled a mental health streaming area designed to provide specialised assessment for patients in a mental health crisis when they attended the accident and emergency department. However, we had received concerns about patient safety due to extended length of stays for patients in the streaming area during times of operational pressure when demand exceeded capacity.

As this was a trial involving collaboration between two Trusts with two separate cultures and specialties, we felt it was crucial to ask the staff involved in the patient's care what had happened due to the extended length of stay in the streaming area.

I had conducted AARs before for the Trust and found them to be an incredibly powerful tool to assess the contributory factors involved in adverse events. It also regularly helped to empower staff to be part of any change identified. I suggested we conducted an AAR across the two Trusts.

### What We Did

I initially approached the senior leads from both Trusts who had both raised concerns and wanted to see improvement within the service. I explained to the senior leads what AAR was and what it aimed to achieve and asked them to lead in approaching the relevant staff involved. I also explained to them that the AAR recommendations made by staff would then need to be heard and honoured to see any cultural change between the services. Both the senior leads were open to the approach and happy to facilitate the review.

The Director of Nursing for my division and the Senior Operational Manager at the Mental Health Trust were instrumental in coordinating the AAR. They shared the AAR guidance with the staff and explained that they wanted to create a safe space for staff to be heard in a non-hierarchical process. We decided to do a virtual AAR because the staff members were based in different Trust sites and also because of the number of staff potentially involved.

Although 19 staff members were identified as having delivered care to the patient, we expected some hesitation in attending the virtual AAR as it was a first for many of the staff; however, 15 staff members in total attended, representing many roles at different levels, including healthcare assistants, registered nurses, chaplains, operational managers, matrons and advanced care practitioners.

I was initially nervous about how to keep focus in a virtual forum with so many staff from different services. An AAR needs a certain level of concentration and for the AAR Conductor to provide space for every staff member to have a voice.

I explained the scope of the exercise — that this was not a punitive process but a learning review and asked for respect and process-driven language rather than language directed at individuals or teams.

At first, there were members of the group who seemed to be uncomfortable with the process, giving monosyllabic answers or being hesitant to talk. I could sense that individuals deeply wanted to respond or react to other's experiences of the event and at some stages had raised their hands to respond to other people's experiences. I asked for members of the AAR to hear all experiences and allow this to be used as group reflection as well as acknowledging what their experience was.

## What Actually Happened

The engagement from the staff was incredible. Although there had clearly been evidence of strained relationships between teams at times, during the AAR it became clear that all had shared a common goal to want to deliver the best care for their patients. Everyone had psychologically safe, controlled and maintained time to talk and share their experience of the patient journey and all could offer valid recommendations.

We explained at the start that we would take notes to capture the actions and made it clear that we had no plans to record the AAR or take individual staff members' names as this was a safe space. This seemed to put people at ease.

As we progressed, the group became more open to the process and felt more relaxed and comfortable. The members of the review gave more detailed answers and reflected on others' experiences. At one point, a senior operational manager noted how touched he was that at the heart of all the experiences described, the staff were focused on the patient's best interests.

## Lessons Learned

One tip I would give to others conducting an AAR is to expect some resistance from staff who have perhaps only witnessed punitive processes regarding incidents or events. Do not be disheartened when the world does not change overnight from one AAR. With any good learning tool, it is one of many in your armoury. For me, it is a powerful one that is the most person-centred and holistic.

Next time, I would identify one senior lead to take forward the recommendations so staff know that their voices will be heard. I would also identify beforehand one governance forum to review the findings of the AAR. I would recommend, if possible, conducting an AAR face to face, with a maximum of 5 or 6 key staff members to keep it focused without staff losing interest — although I would never turn interested relevant parties away.

## Evaluation and Impact

Staff members described why there was a difference between what was expected to happen and what actually happened and there was useful insight into the situation that could be built into recommendations. Suggestions were made focusing on improvements in shared pathways, culture, communication, information systems and escalation systems. The notes were typed up and shared with the group to comment on. With full agreement from the group, these were then shared with the senior leads.

Afterwards, I collected informal feedback about the AAR from staff; there was reluctance to involve a more formal feedback structure as AAR was still in its infancy and I wanted to ensure that it was seen as user friendly and not 'wrapped up in red tape'.

The informal feedback was positive from staff members from both Trusts:

'I felt that this was the first time the teams had talked together about what had happened.'

'I could feel that I wanted to respond straight away at first to what other staff members had shared, but because there was controlled space between their experience and the next, it gave me time to reflect and review.'

A senior lead said that he 'was comforted that all the concerns raised were because the teams wanted to deliver the right care to the patient.'

Since this AAR, the AAR process has commenced throughout the Trust in pockets of excellent work. I think the process could be improved by having a formal structure in place for AAR feedback so it can provide a bigger impact.

Currently, in many Trusts, it is viewed as something that is 'nice to do' instead of incredibly relevant information to improve patient and staff outcomes for the better. The next step is to embed it into the governance structure through the PSIRF framework. The governance leads are setting this as one of the priorities to promote shared learning.

## Conclusions

I think there is scope for AAR training to be delivered for all senior leaders and staff teams in hospitals. I have a regular senior team meeting and try to take an opportunity once a month to ask: 'what was expected to happen compared to what actually happened'. I have also suggested to matrons and ward leaders that this can be done in an informal way at the end of a shift to help staff in debrief.

Although I had great hopes that big changes would be made directly from the AAR, I must acknowledge that this was carried out in a period where we are under extreme operational pressure within the NHS. The AAR was shared with the staff involved in it and the mental health streaming area monitored closely for any other patient safety issues. The two Trusts have had joint meetings to discuss the differing information systems and shared details of risks identified and started to progress in joint investigations around patient care.

A shared learning forum was identified from one of the recommendations of the AAR to improve communication across the two Trusts and work further on embedding a culture of learning. This shared learning forum has been designed and an anonymised copy of the AAR recommendations will be the first agenda item of the forum.

### CASE STUDY 2

Lisa Moss, Acute Hospital Trust

## Background

A medication safety incident was reported to the local incident reporting system and initially was graded Amber with moderate harm. It involved a patient on a medical ward that had been administered double the dose of analgesia that had been prescribed to her. This analgesia was a controlled drug.

This level of harm would initiate a Duty of Candour and the level of grading would have indicated an RCA to be carried out. However, following review, it was felt that the level of harm could be reduced; therefore, professional Duty of Candour became applicable. The grading of this incident remained Amber as it was felt there was an opportunity for learning.

We decided to use the AAR methodology to review this incident. We chose to use AAR as it was felt that the simplicity of the template would highlight the areas of learning and, as an organisation transitioning from the Serious Incident Framework (SIF) to PSIRF, this was one of the very first methodologies that the team was trialling in an attempt to move away from RCA.

We hoped by completing an AAR, the team would very quickly, with minimal time and effort, identify what happened and why, and highlight the system vulnerabilities that led to this incident occurring.

I was keen to use the AAR template and incorporate the systems methodology SEIPS into the discussion and write up of the incident.

This would formulate the learning and recommendations for safety.

## What We Did

Once alerted to the incident via the trust incident reporting system, the patient safety lead emailed the ward manager and matron for the area with a proposal to move away from RCA and to use AAR. Initially this was met with some trepidation as the language was very new and both the ward manager and the matron were unsure of how to proceed.

We gave them the AAR template along with the NHS ACT Academy 'After Action Review' information (NHS England, 2021) and a proposal to meet with them and the nursing team to facilitate the discussion. At this point the most senior nurse involved was the matron for the area.

A meeting date and time was set, and two patient safety leads went to the ward area to meet with the staff. The meeting was in the patients' day room on the medical ward as it was quiet so there would be no interruptions during the meeting. Seven staff attended the meeting: the matron, the ward manager, a Band 6 nurse on duty at the time, the two nurses involved in the incident and the two patient safety leads.

With everyone gathered it became apparent that the two nurses involved were very nervous and clearly felt under pressure. With more senior staff attending it may have appeared as if they were walking into a disciplinary meeting. We all sat in a circle to ensure there was no feeling of hierarchy and gave introductions to make the atmosphere feel relaxed and light-hearted. We set the scene very quickly:

- We explained who we were.
- We explained a little about SIF and how PSIRF is very different as the nurses knew very little about either process.
- We reassured them that this was not a punitive process but one that was about understanding what had happened and how we would, as a team, put in place mechanisms to prevent such incidents happening again.
- That they should not worry, the focus was entirely on learning and development and did not in any way represent a disciplinary process.

Once we had set the scene, we discussed the incident and asked them in their own words to tell us what their version of events were. Again, we explained that the discussion was for learning purposes, and we highlighted that healthcare is a very complex system and to understand the complexities we needed to understand what had happened.

We discussed good practice and discussed in a collaborative way recommendations for improvement.

## Lessons Learned

Both patient safety leads had little experience with completing AARs but were experienced nurses. What surprised them was the level of anxiety from the staff present.

Setting the scene prior to the meeting is crucial to ensure that everyone is fully aware that AARs are about learning and not holding people to account to minimise staff distress.

The two nurses involved were internationally educated nurses, and from their body language and from their discussion it was apparent that they believed that they were in trouble and were going to be either disciplined or reported to their governing body. This highlighted that the current culture has a potential to focus on blame and is something that needs to be addressed throughout the organisation.

We explained this was not the case and explained just culture and they did relax a little, but it was not a good start to the review. This is something that should be taken into consideration for subsequent AARs.

A barrier to communication may have been because the patient safety leads were in matron uniforms, which may have exacerbated the feeling of a top-heavy approach in the room.

When the AAR was concluded, the patient safety leads spent further time with those at the meeting to 'chat' about their day-to-day job, the difficulties and the challenges. We felt it was important to be relaxed and to try to reduce the stress that this AAR potentially caused the group.

We chatted about their careers and their home life, again to diffuse any anxiety. Going forward this is not something that we feel we will need to continue to do but for this first AAR, for both the patient safety leads and the staff, it was something that we felt was appropriate.

For this case, we were able to meet with the staff easily soon after the event, but this may not always be possible. Gathering staff who work shifts can delay the timing of the AAR and work pressures within the Trust is another challenge to meeting with staff in a time-sensitive way.

As with every new process, you learn from what went well and what did not go so well and get better at the process with time and experience.

## Evaluation and Impact

Overall, the AAR process was well-received. It was felt that this way forward would achieve a better outcome — enhancing patients' safety, and for those staff involved in an incident, a positive experience that they could learn from in a safe non-challenging way. Feedback from staff overall was positive.

One staff member said that she was very anxious at the start but afterwards felt that she had learnt and felt positive if she was ever required to take part in the process again. It made her feel part of the team and that they were all working together to help each other and improve the safety for the patients.

As it was the first AAR that we had facilitated it did not go as smoothly as anticipated. Going forward it may be something that the patient safety team would want to simulate to ensure the process was as well led as possible. It was felt that this was key to ensuring the staff benefited from the process as much as possible.

The executive team were anxious on how any safety recommendations that were captured would be actioned and monitored. AAR used initially by the US army in the field on combat missions can demonstrate changes straight away and, arguably, do not need to be evidenced. This is not the case for AARs completed for patient safety incidents.

We have yet to agree how to monitor the recommendations going forward in this Trust.

We want to avoid safety recommendations sitting in silo in local areas and for learning to be disseminated widely so that others can learn. We also want to ensure that the AAR is not a paper exercise and is more effective than the RCAs have been.

## Conclusions

Following completion of this AAR we reflected on what went well and what did not go so well. We learned that it is important to be well prepared and to have skills in facilitation to ensure the smooth running of the review. Overall, the process has considerable benefits over the RCA methodology: it is faster, the learning can be put into place immediately and there is wider staff involvement.

PSIRF promotes 'Patient Safety is everyone's business' and involving staff right at the centre of the incident will promote this ethos.

## Reflections from the Frontline

- In both the case studies, staff had not undertaken any formal AAR training. The AARs have been undertaken as a 'trial' with the staff researching the principles of AAR online and attending patient safety forums. As we progress, AARs will be carried out by different staff with different roles, different levels of seniority and within different settings. To train every member of staff within healthcare by an affiliated AAR provider will not be possible due to time and financial constraints. A 'train the trainer' approach may be a solution; however, this runs the risk of knowledge being 'watered down'.
- The role of the AAR Conductor has not been fully understood. Careful facilitation of the AAR is crucial, and training in the facilitation and principles of AAR needs to be undertaken to enable everyone to be heard and group learning to be identified. It may be unrealistic to source a Conductor outside of the incident environment, especially out of hours. In reality, the Conductor will usually be a clinician on the ward/department, and this may introduce bias.
- MDTs and the complexity of differing shift patterns and rotas may make getting the original staff who were involved in an incident together for the AAR difficult. However, if it is only the nursing team, for example, that is the only constant in an incident, then there is the risk that the AAR will only gain one perspective and medical opinion or input from other areas will be missing, leading to inadequate recommendations and silo working.
- Staff who are unclear of the AAR process may have misunderstandings, such as 'recommendations do not need to be documented or evidenced' or 'AAR must happen as soon as possible after the event'. These misunderstandings may lead to the AAR being rushed and recommendations not being recorded.

- Governance teams during the transition into PSIRF may require additional information; this then may create a lengthy document which may resemble a root cause analysis. These habits may then be difficult to break.
- When patients and families are informed of the outcomes of an AAR and the actions arising as a result, some of the first victim information needs will be met. This is certainly the experience of a number of NHS Trusts that have initiated this practice already. When patients are invited to contribute to the AARs themselves, the level of transparency is significantly increased and the potential for understanding and forgiveness is, therefore, much higher. At present, the capability and confidence of staff to undertake an AAR with family and patient present will need to be addressed with sufficient training, peer support and guidance.

## References

Carayon P. *et al*. (2006). 'Work system design for patient safety: the SEIPS model' in *Quality Safety Health Care*, 15(Suppl 1): pp. i50–i58.

Crowe, J. *et al*. (2017). 'After-action reviews: The good behaviour, the bad behavior, and why we should care' in *Safety Science*, 96: pp. 84–92.

Darling, M., Parry, C. and Moore, J. (2005). 'Learning in the Thick of It' in *Harvard Business Review*, 83(7): pp. 84–92.

Dekker, S. (2014). *The Field Guide to Understanding 'Human Error'*. Oxfordshire: Routledge.

Edmondson, A. (1999). 'Psychological Safety and Learning Behaviour in Work Teams' in *Administrative Science Quarterly*, 44(2): pp. 350–383.

General Medical Council (2019). *Benefits of becoming a reflective practitioner*. https://www.gmc-uk.org/education/standards-guidance-and-curricula/guidance/reflective-practice/benefits-of-becoming-a-reflective-practitioner.

General Medical Council of United Kingdom — Ethical Guidance for doctors. The Professional Duty of Candour. Online. https://www.gmc-uk.org/professional-standards/professional-standards-for-doctors/candour---openness-and-honesty-when-things-go-wrong/the-professional-duty-of-candour#:~:text=Every%20health%20and%20care%20professional,to%20cause%2C%20harm%20or%20distress.

Kahneman, D. (2012). *Thinking, Fast and Slow*. London: Penguin.

Knowles, M.S. *et al*. (1984). *Andragogy in action: Applying modern principles of adult education*. San Francisco: Jossey-Bass.

Kolb, D.A. (1984). *Experiential Learning: Experience as the Source of Learning and Development*. New Jersey: Prentice-Hall.

Kolbe, M. *et al*. (2021). 'Team debriefings in healthcare: aligning intention and impact' in *BMJ*, 374:n2042.

Kumar, M. (2023). *Team Based Quality Review*. RCSEd, NHS Education Scotland. Online: www.rcsed.ac.uk/news-public-affairs/the-rcsed-blog/2023/september/team-based-quality-reviews.

Morrison, J.E. and Meliza, L.L. (1999). 'The Foundations of the After Action Review Process' in *United States Army Research Institute for the Behavioral and Social Sciences Special Report 42*.

NHS England (2021). *Online library of Quality, Service Improvement and Redesign tools: After Action Review*. Online. https://aqua.nhs.uk/QSIR/.

Nursing and Midwifery Council of United Kingdon (NMC) (2015). *The Code: Professional standards of practice and behaviour for nurses, midwives and nursing associates*. Online. https://www.nmc.org.uk/standards/code/.

Pascale, R., Milleman, M. and Gioja, L. (2001). *Surfing the Edge of Chaos: The Laws of Nature and the New Laws of Business*. New York: Crown Publishing.

Renshaw, M., Tucker, P. and Norman, K. (2020). 'Becoming fall-safe: a framework for reducing inpatient falls' in *British Journal of Nursing*, 29(20): pp. 1198–1205.

Salter, M.S. and Klein, G.E. (2007). *After Action Reviews: Current Observations and Recommendations U.S. Army Research Institute for the Behavioral and Social Sciences*. Vienna, VA: The Wexford Group International, Inc.

Tannenbaum, S.I. and Cerasoli, C.P. (2013). 'Do team and individual debriefs enhance performance? A meta-analysis'. *Journal of Human Factors*, Feb; 55(1): pp. 231–45.

Walker, J. *et al*. (2012). 'Life in the slow lane: making hospitals safer, slowly but surely' in *Journal of the Royal Society of Medicine*, 105(7): pp. 283–7.

# CHAPTER 7

# Walk-Through-Talk-Through Analysis to Support Healthcare Safety and Improvement Activity

*Richard Brownhill and Paul Bowie*

## Summary

This chapter outlines basic guidance on how those working in healthcare can apply a Human Factors informed systems approach using Walk-Through-Talk-Through (WT3) to understand, evaluate and improve human work. More specifically it sets out to:

1. Describe and outline guiding steps in applying the WT3 process.
2. Outline the importance of exploring system-wide performance influencing factors (PIFs) when evaluating aspects of human work.
3. Introduce the *In Situ* Structured Observation Guide (I-SOG) as a practical data collection template and question set to aid users when applying the WT3 process.
4. Illustrate the application of WT3 via a small number of short case studies across different care sectors.

The chapter will inform some of your approach and thinking in relation to observation, examining its implications, context, and potential considerations. Although there are several methods, it presents a relatively practical and applied tool for everyday work analysis.

## Background

Observing and interacting with the activities of people are used by all of us formally and informally every day of our lives; for example, considering the gap needed to cross the road, monitoring our children brushing their teeth or listening to an announcement at the station. We rapidly interpret what we hear, ask, see and sense, and use the analysis of this raw data to provide us with information with which to inform how these activities are performed and what to do next.

One useful approach widely applied in the field of Human Factors and Ergonomics (HFE) is WT3 analysis. This is a formal, structured approach to collecting data through interacting *in situ* with people performing work, asking probing questions about these activities, listening carefully to what is said and by whom, and observing what is done and how it is done. In healthcare quality and safety activity, this type of method is underused but has great potential and is, arguably, foundational and necessary in determining how everyday work is really done to better inform the design of improvement interventions and 'solutions'; i.e. capturing, comparing and reconciling 'work as imagined' and 'work as done'. Addressing differences in these two work principles is a key element fundamental to the HFE discipline, where the adoption of a holistic 'systems approach' to understand the dynamic and interactive nature of complex sociotechnical work systems more adequately is core (Hollnagel and Clay-Williams,

2022). However, we do not appear to have a shared understanding of what this entails in healthcare, nor is it routinely and explicitly apparent in how we undertake patient safety and QI activity.

Seeking to embed HFE thinking and tools within patient safety, QI, risk control and educational activities is one way to promote progress, but also to demonstrate examples of the basic principles adopted by the science (e.g. the systems approach) to better aid understanding and lessen confusion and misinterpretation in healthcare.

In a comparative review of ten HFE methods that could be performed by non-specialist, novice users, both *observation* and *interviews* were considered potentially more feasible data collection and analysis methods than other more challenging HFE techniques, where it was recommended that greater caution should be exercised as more in-depth training would be necessary.

## What is WT3?

WT3 is a combined verbal walkthrough analysis and observation tool. From a healthcare safety and improvement perspective, it can be used to collect and analyse data about a task or activity (e.g. taking a blood sample from a patient), scenario (e.g. a specific patient safety incident) or future development (e.g. designing a vaccination programme). It is undertaken to aid comprehension of how work is or will be performed in 'real world' settings. Important reasons for applying a WT3 are that it can, for example, be used as part of a prospective hazard identification process, to inform design of work procedures, or to help to identify error-producing conditions, everyday work hassles, frustrations and irritations (and the PIFs that increase their likelihood or make work unnecessarily complex or confusing). Significantly, we can also learn how frontline teams can adapt to recover from related situations and introduce rapid work improvements that further support and enhance both human performance and overall system functioning. It is worth noting that this differs from, for example, a leadership walk-round which is a more generalised and unstructured process of actively listening to staff concerns about work. The WT3 is applied to examine or evaluate a specific, defined work task, scenario or situation with a view to informing redesign and/or improvement.

WT3 is one of a group of similar, overlapping methods (e.g. cognitive walkthrough, Norman cognitive walkthrough, heuristic walkthrough, think-aloud technique) often used to understand and evaluate different types of work systems, such as the usability of digital technology or job tasks performed by frontline operators. It is commonly used by HFE specialists as one way to better understand how 'everyday work is actually done' in real-time by those at the 'sharp-end' of practice and is especially useful as part of a formal task analysis. In this way, by seeking multiple verbalised perspectives from team members on how tasks are performed combined with observations of work *in situ*, more informative and contextualised improvement and system redesign needs can potentially be uncovered. For example, WT3 can facilitate diverse conversations and understandings around the value and relevance of work procedures (e.g. clinical protocols), the necessary trade-offs and adaptations to work that are required, and the role of technology or the prevailing safety culture and how these interact to influence human and overall system performance. Mastering and embedding this 'simple' approach can potentially add value to our patient safety, QI and risk control activities — and make a useful and important contribution to the integration of HFE principles and approaches within this work.

## Anticipated Benefits of WT3

Operational healthcare teams working at the 'sharp end' (especially those in direct contact with patients) experience mixed exposure to patient safety and QI teams, often premised on the maturity of an organisation's safety culture and approaches to learning. As clinical care is highly complex, observation as a single perspective cannot evaluate the competence or risks of a particular activity in the absence of a description, dialogue or narrative. So unwittingly purposing people to go and 'look' or observe something would be a futile task. Using experiences from improvement work, it is common to work alongside a team you haven't met before, sharing a common desire to 'make things better'. To make contact and work with teams proactively as well as to build trust is a strong element of getting deep and meaningful insights to inform thinking, perspectives and improvement aims. Knowing what outputs people are trying to achieve helps to provide a boundary as to what to explore, otherwise we risk being overwhelmed, distracted or having an unstructured foray into a service/task.

Through observation, the benefits of sharing insights appear to develop mutual trust, shared understanding and learning. There may be common oversimplifications of what we think happens in settings and circumstances meaning we may not appreciate risks, trade-offs, or workarounds that staff have to do to help keep themselves and their patients safe.

Proactive safety conversations and visits by safety teams can also offer the psychological safety and support to help identify and amplify safety concerns. Examining where the work takes place, when, by whom, capturing multiple perspectives, and sharing insights can help to drive safety culture within the service/clinical area as well as spreading rationale and understanding more widely.

It may go without saying that it is a courtesy to introduce who we are or what department we are from, but, beyond this, the conversation may best be reflected in sharing that you are 'here to help'. You are trying to understand what would make things better, you are there to listen, you are there to see what really happens and often how tricky it is to balance many, often conflicting, priorities and do the difficult work that is associated with healthcare. This may appear daunting to some as you may find yourself in an unfamiliar environment with little knowledge or understanding of where you are or what goes on. However, the opportunity can be used to also consider the experience from a new staff or patient perspective and what quickly orientates you (e.g. signage, environment, user-based design). There may be a requirement to have relevant personal protective equipment or undergo an information briefing before you begin a period of observation. The surprise of finding yourself standing in an operating theatre for six hours may challenge any of us without adequate preparation. It does highlight that this would influence how those working in this environment are able to remain at their optimal (e.g. hydrated, comfortable, attentive). Many teams are likely to tell you 'how things are' and recognise/invite the value of your perspective, so adopting a flexible approach is key. It's a conversation, a safety or improvement discussion but nonetheless a skill that requires tenacity, compassion, the ability to listen and to clarify.

A knowledge of Human Factors can make observation more potent, and while formal HFE education among healthcare staff remains slower than other complex industries, access to 'simpler' HFE methods for novice users can provide support in conjunction with guidance, training and feedback. An example of this is the iSOG tool in Appendix 1, which offers a structured framework to help to guide observation and understanding of tasks.

## Performance Influencing Factors (PIFs)

It is important at the outset to understand the role of PIFs and identify and explore the presence of these conditions as part of the WT3 process and how they shape success or hinder it. PIFs refer to both immediate and latent (background) work conditions that can influence human and wider work system performance and contribute to process difficulty (e.g. overly complex tasks or inadequately designed work procedures), or directly to unwanted outcomes such as patient safety incidents or staff burnout issues.

Table 7.1 outlines examples and explanations of the potential role of PIFs. Each PIF grouping is aligned with the six interacting work systems elements that form part of the SEIPS framework: people, tasks, tools and technology, physical environment, organisations and external factors. SEIPS is a well-established Human Factors framework that has been used as a flexible work systems analysis method in multiple studies across healthcare sectors internationally (see Chapter 3 on SEIPS).

**Table 7.1** Examples of Systems-Wide Performance Influencing Factors (PIFs)

| SEIPS System Element | Performance Influencing Factor | Explanation/Examples |
|---|---|---|
| **People** | *Personal* | • Personal factors influencing performance may vary over time and are individual to a person, but may include stress, low morale, boredom, lack of confidence or complacency, poor mental or physical health (including chronic or acute fatigue), being under the influence of drugs or alcohol or otherwise impaired, etc. |
| | *Training and experience* | • Task performance can be adversely affected by a lack of familiarity with a task or inadequate experience of performing a task, poor training or mentoring quality, a lack of training or a time gap between training and doing the task, and/or a lack of opportunity to develop sufficient competence. |
| **Task** | *Task* | • Task factors are related to excessive demands of the task, excessively high (or low) workload, competing tasks, working under time pressure, complex tasks demanding high levels of concentration, tasks that demand good visibility, dexterity or are physically demanding, tasks that are very monotonous and repetitive, situations with many distractions, interruptions or divided attention, or non-standard activities. |
| **Tools and technology** | *Human-technology interaction and design* | • The equipment that people interact with, the conditions of that interaction or factors in workspace design can induce failure. Examples of technological PFIs include poorly presented information or a lack of information, too much automation, poor quality alarms or alarm overload, poor equipment positioning, poor quality or reliability of equipment, inappropriate work tools for the task, unclear signs and signals, inadequate workplace access or workspace arrangement, or tools that make the task more difficult, such as personal protective equipment. |
| | *Design of work procedures* | • Procedures or work instructions can make error more likely through being absent or highly variable in task method, or by being inaccurate, poorly presented, unintelligible, overly complex and/or ambiguous or unclear. |
| **Physical environment** | *Ambient environment* | • The ambient environment can present significant challenges to performance and may include the weather, thermal environment, lighting, noise, air quality and/or the presence of health hazards. These interact strongly with the reliability of tasks — see task factors, stress and fatigue, and see personal factors. |
| | *Workplace design* | • Workplace designs e.g. in room or department layout that fail to consider human limitations, needs and capabilities can introduce risks that impact on the physical and psychological well-being of the workforce, which in turn affects performance and productivity. |

| SEIPS System Element | Performance Influencing Factor | Explanation/Examples |
|---|---|---|
| Organisational | Communication<br><br>Social and team<br><br>Leadership<br><br>Supervision<br><br>Culture | • Communication (information flow) is a vital organisational influence on performance and outcomes and can be verbal, nonverbal or written (including electronic). PIFs include high communications workload, poor phrasing or low communication standards, language/dialectical differences, the content of the information, the quality and method of communication (and the reliability/quality of interacting communications equipment).<br>• Social and team factors may include issues affecting teamwork, such as difficult relationships and team dynamics, sub-optimal coordination and/or a lack of team maturity. PIFs also include inadequately defined roles and responsibilities, work scheduling, staffing levels and poor shift handover, as well as poor supervision, poor safety culture and a lack of focus on organisational factors during the management of change. |
| External | External | • External factors that can impact on how human work is done in frontline practice may include national targets, policy and regulatory demands, accreditation standards, political decision making and global events. |

## Exploring Human Work

As stated, a key principle within HFE is the notion of 'work as imagined' versus 'work as done'. The WT3 method offers a real time opportunity to have individuals/teams describe the tasks they do. Developing the description through narrative ('work-as-described' through those at the 'sharp-end') and visual representation ('work-as-prescribed' in rules and policies), the WT3 method then moves on to observe and capture what takes place (in the moment) but with the opportunity to clarify individual rationale/thinking as the task happens. Some of the insights offered then enable timely feedback discussions and opportunities to offer suggestions to build for further exploration, development and improvement.

# How to Apply WT3

Stanton *et al.* (2013) suggest that there are no set rules for WT3, but have suggested some basic guiding steps that have been adapted here for the healthcare context:

**Step 1. Define the task, scenario or activity**
The task(s) or scenario for the system under analysis should be defined and be representative of the work undertaken. The people involved in the related work should also be defined and representatives of the system users should participate in the WT3 analysis.

**Step 2. Visually describe the task, scenario or activity**
Once defined, the task, scenario or activity would benefit from being described so that the different component parts are clearer and simpler to understand, ideally using a visual tool such as Hierarchical Task Analysis (HTA) or simple process mapping. For novice users, HTA is likely to be a more complex and challenging process and will require some training and practice, whereas process mapping is arguably a simpler and more easily accessible tool, especially with access to basic guidance. Indeed, some of the limitations of process mapping in complex

care systems are arguably overcome by effective, complementary use of WT3. Depending on feasibility or the study context, Step 2 can potentially be skipped and undertaken as part of Step 3.

**Step 3. Perform WT3**
A dedicated WT3 lead should perform a simple verbalised walkthrough of the relevant work system design in conjunction with, where possible, multiple system users reflective of the workforce. The process can be stopped at any time to: ask questions when observing tasks; review documentation, devices or decisions being made; or to seek more detailed clarity on social, technological or organisational aspects of the task or scenario. Ideally the WT3 should be recorded using a recording device (sound or video where feasible) and/or contemporaneous notes taken by the lead analyst using a standardised systems-based template such as the I-SOG (Morgan & Bowie, 2020; Appendix 1). Problems with the system design (e.g. hazards encountered, error-producing conditions identified, unused or inadequate work procedures) should be noted as potential improvement opportunities.

**Step 4. Analyse data**
WT3 data are flexible and may be qualitative (e.g. recorded notes on the adequacy of clinical guidelines or observations of peoples' actions and behaviours) or quantitative (e.g. task frequency, number of hazards identified, reported incidents, improvement targets) or a mix of both. The data from different sources should be triangulated, analysed appropriately and interpreted in line with the study purpose to increase validity and credibility. The resulting information can be used for multiple purposes, for example: to propose new or redesigned risk controls; modify existing work procedures to make them more usable; make a safety case or argument for a way of working; streamline steps in a set of work tasks as part of a safety audit; or inform design of a QI or implementation project.

**Step 5. Improve work system design**
The work system design can be modified as agreed based on the problems and potential solutions identified. However, where this happens a further WT3 should be conducted to evaluate the impact of the (re-)design. Similarly, system change may also be enhanced using formal rapid Plan, Do, Study, Act (PDSA) cycles to support the improvement process on an iterative basis.

## Who Can Use WT3?

WT3 has both multi-functional and multi-user potential in healthcare to understand how human work is really done. Any healthcare worker or educator can lead and apply the implementation of the WT3 process in collaboration with colleagues who typically perform the work-related task, scenario or activity being evaluated, regardless of whether it is seen as safety-critical, highly complex, problematic or simple. For example, it could be of interest to the following workforce groups:

- For clinical risk, patient safety and quality improvement advisors it should be a fundamental approach that can be deployed when working alongside clinical and non-clinical teams to initially explore and better understand how different aspects of human work are undertaken as part of QI, safety or service redesign projects.
- For safety investigators, WT3 may have a very specific role as part of post-incident learning investigations where it can be applied *in situ* when visiting healthcare facilities to jointly examine with clinical teams how routine work normally goes well but can sometimes go wrong.
- For clinicians-in-training WT3 can be applied, with the support of brief practical guidance, as part of QI activity, induction or personal development, and established clinical teams can use it as part of local service evaluations and improvement.

- Health services researchers may also adapt the method as part of ethnographic observational studies of frontline clinical practices, particularly for those with a focus on patient safety or workforce well-being.
- Finally, clinical educators may wish to consider the need to include this type of method as part of training curricula, and in both designing or debriefing clinical simulation scenarios, given its foundational importance in exploring patient safety and quality improvement issues.

Boxes 7.1 and 7.2 show examples of how and where WT3 can be used.

> **BOX 7.1** Example of WT3 Used in an Acute Hospital
>
> WT3 was used in the investigation of a blood sampling incident. The investigators first reviewed local blood sampling policies and then asked nursing staff to perform a series of mock blood samples. This involved shadowing the nurses as they created the request, collected equipment, visited the bedside, labelled the sample and sent the sample for testing. The investigators asked questions to clarify why certain actions were completed at each stage of the process. WT3 identified a gap between work as imagined and work as done. Staff had adapted their practice to account for the layout of the local ward environment which made it impractical to follow the steps prescribed in the blood sampling policy. This prompted a review to identify whether redesigning the ward environment could facilitate safer blood sampling practice.

> **BOX 7.2** Example of WT3 Used in a Dental Setting
>
> WT3 was used as a learning investigation following a near-miss incident involving contaminated instruments potentially being used on a patient. This incorporated the In Situ Structured Observation Guide (I-SOG) as a template. The decontamination procedures and policies were initially reviewed followed by shadowing of the nurse and dentist through a variety of simulated typical tasks involving instrument changeover and decontamination prior to treating the next patient. The investigator asked questions of both clinicians and nurses to understand why each action was necessary at the time and the reason for any adaptations that were being made. WT3 revealed deeper organisational factors and a gap between work as imagined and work as done. Adaptations by frontline staff were being made due to time pressures in patient scheduling and a lack of breaks and staff training. This highlighted the need for further analysis of work as done to inform the redesign of work schedules, decontamination processes and training to decrease worker fatigue and increase patient safety.

## Key Questions and Prompts

When applying WT3, the related I-SOG template (Appendix 1) has been designed to help facilitate necessary conversations with colleagues when evaluating the task, scenario, or activity of interest, and when taking contemporaneous notes, sketches or even uploading photographs (with consent) of task-related activity. The overall goal here is to understand and close the gap between work as imagined and work as done. Work as imagined refers to the assumptions underpinning work rules, regulations and guidance, and which often resides in the minds of those removed from sharp-end practice (e.g. leaders and policymakers). In this perspective, work tasks can be comprehensively analysed and prescribed — this is an idealised but unrealistic view of how work is performed in highly complex sociotechnical systems. Work as done, however, describes the reality of how everyday work actually occurs and how people performing tasks must routinely adjust what they do to match the everchanging conditions and demands of work. The key point here is that complex work systems are successful most of the time because the workforce is generally adaptive and flexible to the changing conditions of work as done, not because systems of work have been expertly designed or because people always follow the recommended guidance to the letter (work as imagined). The WT3 process enables all of these issues to be explored with a view to closing the gap between work as imagined and work as done and so better support human work performance.

## Advantages and Disadvantages of WT3

The main advantages of the WT3 process are that it can be conducted without technical equipment or infrastructure, except people. Whilst it requires little training for the most part and is relatively simple, quick and low cost, knowledge and experience of HFE will enhance its application/interpretation. Importantly, it has the potential to provide a detailed and accurate description of the task or scenario under analysis and offer design or redesign proposals to improve the work system. The WT3 process can be used as a single intervention or dovetail with other patient safety and QI methods. Importantly, it can be incorporated as part of clinical simulation scenarios as a training intervention or to examine a process or plan for a new service.

Some reported disadvantages include the need to have access to team member(s) experienced in the task or scenario, while the reliability of the technique and the need for guidance on preparation and analysis are also questioned. Evidence of its routine use and impact in supporting patient safety and QI project activity is also limited.

As with all methods, individuals may bring their own biases to bear as part of what we see, hear, and interpret. To assist with this, we can triangulate with other data (e.g. reports, measures), engage in more interaction to understand more richly, and reflect personally on whether we consider what we are interpreting as justifiable.

## Other Considerations

There may be concerns, thoughts or opinions that when we observe/interact with teams they may somehow alter or change their behaviour, often considered in research as the Hawthorne effect (Sedgwick and Greenwood, 2015). This originates from an increased productivity seen when a group of workers were intensively supervised in a telecoms factory in the 1920s/30s. McCambridge *et al.* (2014), in a systematic review, suggested that whilst some evidence of an effect appears to exist, these couldn't easily be identified or understood. Acquiescence bias is reported in research where favourable responses are offered by participants to please the researcher (Bowling, 2014).

The degree to which people are changing or modifying behaviour as part of a walkthrough is of interest to those in HFE/patient safety, not because it may in some way be deceptive or deliberate, rather it may identify the sense of a hierarchy gradient or may be a barometer of psychological safety within systems.

## Final Thoughts

Observation walkthrough will remain an important feature of seeing 'work as done' rather than 'work as imagined', though ensuring we seek the critical insights of those undertaking the task will help to provide understanding and rationale about what behaviours, approaches and adaptations make sense. As observation is just one input when considering a complex situation, it is best conducted combined with additional data sources, responses, surveys, images, interviews, and the perspectives of other stakeholders.

In using this method, we may inadvertently invoke a hierarchy gradient, bring hindsight or cognitive bias to the situation yet strengthen safety culture. Adopting the WT3 process as a widely used tool in Human Factors aids understanding and analysis of how work is done, though this combined verbal walkthrough analysis and observational method is not formally well established in healthcare despite its potential multi-functional use. It has significant potential to add value to how we currently undertake patient safety and QI project activity and may have similar usefulness in clinical education (e.g. as a tool to support simulation training) and health services research (e.g. as a tool to support ethnographic methods).

Arguably this type of approach should be the first step in any problem-solving activity that attempts to understand and evaluate human work, recognising some training support may be required prior to its application. The evaluation of its use (e.g. face validity, acceptability and feasibility) and its impacts upon learning and improvement need to be determined, although it offers a relatively simple approach (to observers) that should still be of generic interest to those engaged in healthcare safety, improvement, research and related educational activity worldwide.

# Acknowledgements

We are grateful to Dr Lauren Morgan, Deborah Stratford and Deinniol Owens for their contributions to this chapter.

## CASE STUDY 1

Chris Elston and Kayleigh Edwards, Acute Trust

### Background

Observation is part of the PSIRF toolkit, and we wanted to gain a better understanding of observations and how it could be used so it could be taught to others. We didn't set out to use observation for a specific patient safety incident. Instead, we had a student coming in on placement and it seemed an ideal opportunity to get somebody else's point of view who had never seen or used observations. We could then compare our views and what our results were and take it forward. There was no agenda other than to evaluate the tool and to see whether there was a template that we could use.

Based on that, we looked for somewhere to carry out the observation and asked a clinical educator colleague in something completely different if we could use his ward. It was a respiratory ward with 24–28 beds in it, but we only observed in two of the bays.

We decided to observe one nurse doing a medication round as it seemed the most convenient way to get an observation done. The medication round happens multiple times every day and therefore we weren't imposing ourselves on the ward staff too much as it was something they were already doing.

### What We Did

We picked a lunchtime medication round, asked permission of the nurse in charge, and conducted our first observation. However, this was our first mistake. Not knowing anything about it, we'd read the PSIRF documentation and seen a walkthrough template to use. We thought walkthrough and observation were the same thing. But we found out very quickly that it wasn't quite the same thing. The walk-though template is about the frequency that a person uses an item of equipment in a process and how often that process occurs. This was not the information that we were looking for, so therefore the template wasn't what we wanted. So, we reverted to the back of the template, a blank piece of paper, and jotted down notes and drew pictures of where the beds were and the layout of the room. We mapped it out (Figure 7.1) using a spaghetti diagram of where everything was and then the routes people followed.

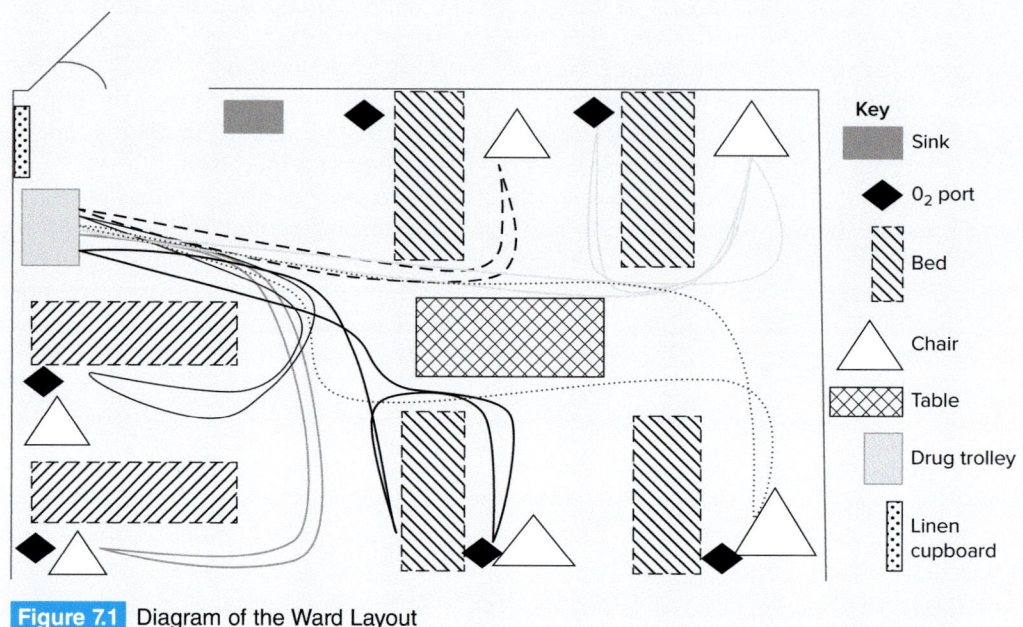

**Figure 7.1** Diagram of the Ward Layout

We spoke to the nurse in charge to say we had permission from the matron to carry out the observation; however, the ward staff had not been told so it was a total surprise to them which wasn't ideal. But we explained to everyone what was happening, and that we weren't looking at elements of their practice but rather that we were evaluating a tool and how it could be used.

One of our concerns when planning the observation was how much we would influence the practice simply by being there — the 'Hawthorne effect' (Sedgwick and Greenwood, 2015) — where you influence something by doing something. However, within a couple of minutes it was evident that our presence had very little impact. We stood to the side, and it was almost as if they just forgot we were there.

Although we hadn't gone into the observation with any specific concerns, there were a few things we did initially pick up by looking at things with a fresh pair of eyes, particularly on the layout of the room. For example, if they would just have had that table over here then it would save the time walking backwards and forwards. Or if they did it in this order it would save on the times they had to walk across to the same spot. But we didn't note anything major.

We stood to one side and watched the first nurse go through the whole process: unlocking the trolley, getting the drugs ready, going to the patient and checking the patient's ID, and administering the medication.

Now, in our minds, you would take the trolley with you to the end of the bed because it's got all your patient safety details on it with the patient's identification on the computer. Instead, they checked the prescription, walked across to the patient, checked the patient's ID wristband against what the patient was saying and then gave them their medication. The reason they did it this way was that there was a huge table in the middle of the room that stopped the drugs trolley from getting down between the table and the bed. So, the nurse obviously made a transaction in their head that rather than negotiate the table and the trolley, they would look at and check the details and keep them fresh in their mind, and then administer medication. We did a spaghetti diagram to show how much of an influence the table played (see Figure 7.1).

We also counted how many times the nurse was interrupted on a drugs round. It is known that the more interruptions you get, the higher the risk of an error. We saw probably about eight or ten interruptions. Simple things like having to move out of the way of the door because of where the drugs trolley was stored. Every time somebody walked into the room or pushed something into the room the nurse had to move out of the way because the drugs trolley was a metre or so away from the door. It was a proper obstruction. It was also situated right next to a linen cupboard so every time somebody had to make a bed, the nurse was also getting interrupted.

That was quite an eye opener because you wouldn't think it would occur so frequently. It's one of those things that if you are doing it every day you just don't see it. It takes a fresh pair of eyes to see it.

## Lessons Learned

### What Worked Well?

It was important for us to do two rooms because as we transited from one room to the other, we came face to face with the drugs trolley going against the bed. The corridor and the passageways are so narrow you can't have both pass each other. And then, when you combine it with the L-shaped ward, the notes trolleys, the drugs trolley and the bed, and several members of staff all trying to pass through the same point at the same time, it was evident that it caused a slight delay and increased the time it takes. It means you have to think a couple of steps ahead of where you are when you are doing something — when going from one room to another you need to think 'will I get through that gap, or do I need to wait?' It's something else to consider which we wouldn't have known about.

When we went into the second room it was a four-bedded bay, with four patients, two drugs trolleys, two nurses administering the drugs, a physiotherapist and two healthcare workers trying to feed patients. You literally couldn't move. It was really crowded, and it brought home just how difficult it is for such a routine task which you don't notice if it's your own clinical area.

We went back a second time and it was useful to observe the second room again. It was less congested this time. We were also told that it would be best to observe a particular nurse as he was the only member of staff that worked there normally. This meant the other staff were less familiar and that showed quickly. We counted 20 interruptions in about 10 minutes, simply because this nurse was the only one that knew where everything was, the layout of the ward and the needs of the patients. It put a huge amount of pressure on this nurse and that was obvious from watching it.

### What Didn't Work so Well?

In hindsight we would have contacted the ward directly to let them know we were coming, which sounds almost counterintuitive as you don't want to prime people that they are being watched in case they changed their practice. However, when we went back up the second time, the nurse in charge didn't know we were coming and as we'd arrived later than the previous occasion, they were a little further advanced in their administration of medications which reduced what we saw.

Going along without a plan was a disadvantage. We knew that we wanted to watch a medication round, but we didn't go along looking for anything in particular. If we had a trigger point — something that had happened that we then went in to evaluate — it would have been a stronger observation than just going along to observe it all.

We did use a template and it was a useful tool because it was laid out in a way that allowed you to make notes about the different Human Factor elements, such as equipment, the environment and the human interactions taking place. However, it's just as easy to go in with a piece of paper and write notes as you see it and put it into a template when you get back to the office. When you've got boxes to tick or certain headings to follow, you maybe miss things as you're so focused on those specific areas.

### Surprises

The one thing that we would say about observations, is that it can be very time consuming. We were on the ward for about 30–45 minutes and we only watched two rooms. If you had a ward which was divided into two teams, and you had full cubicles to look at you could be there for 60–90 minutes.

Probably the biggest surprise was how easy it was to do. Sitting to one side and watching was easier than expected. We picked up a lot and the results we got were more comprehensive than we expected.

Another surprise was how much we wrote down. We had an idea of what we thought we'd be writing down about the process — a step-by-step account of the medication round — but we wrote down so much more than that. We wrote down the issues the layout of the room caused, how many times the nurse had to leave the room to go and get equipment, the interruptions. It surprised us how much there was to it. There was probably much more we missed because we were trying to remain focused on the medication round, but this comes with experience. The more we do the more we'll start to pick up on some of the subtle hints and triggers we're not aware of.

### Tips

Go with a plan. We were very vague and just wanted to evaluate the tool, but we should have focused on evaluating a drugs round. Observations are not something you would want to do without a plan.

If you're doing an observation as a response to a patient safety incident, make sure you're observing the right drugs round or the right things. For example, if the incident happened at 9pm there's no point undertaking an observation at midday as everything is just going to be different.

Do more than one. There's no point observing just one practitioner because we all do it differently. It also then reduces the amount of impact you have so do two, maybe three if you are doing an observation in response to something.

Communicate to those involved. We had good responses, but nobody was expecting us. This might be a good thing if you want to see practice in place and observe how things are done normally but it may not be fair to the ward.

Observe something you don't know in a huge amount of detail. Otherwise, you may focus on whether they're following the right procedures or policies to do the task rather than focusing on the bigger picture.

Watch out for opportunities to expand the observation. This can be an advantage and a disadvantage. On our second day we ended up observing a nurse giving intravenous treatment to a patient. This wasn't our intention, but the nurse ended up doing it as part of the drugs round. It was nice to expand what we were watching but if you are doing a specific investigation into something you have to be very careful not to expand and cover additional things you don't need.

### What Would We do Differently?

We'd like to have had a camera to photograph the layout of the rooms. Trying to describe that second room with the nurse, the physiotherapist, two health care assistants, is difficult in words. A picture would have been far more powerful to show the environment staff are working in and highlight why we need to redesign wards. However, we're not sure that would ever be possible with the rules and regulations around photographing patients and consent.

Time is a big challenge. If we continue with the practice of expecting clinicians to do investigations on top of their normal workload the disadvantage of observations would be the time it takes. This is certainly something that would need a team of investigators to do. It's also useful to have somebody from outside of that clinical environment to do the observation or alongside you if it's your clinical area as they will see it with a fresh pair of eyes. We like the idea of having a non-clinical member of staff, e.g. a porter or a member of the admin staff, as they'll see things that a clinical member may not notice. It would give you a stronger observation and potentially a different focus.

## Evaluation and Impact

We generally had good feedback from staff. However, if you've got a new member staff, who's still learning, you could put a lot of pressure on them by observing them.

It is time consuming but it's offset by the results you get. You will see things that you don't think about back in an office. You don't normally have the opportunity to watch some of the transactions that are being made. Seeing the decision-making process and watching what staff do in order to keep themselves and patients safe against the competing commitments that they've got is so valuable.

We have a PSIRF tools implementation group, and we are looking for patient safety incidents we can use the new tools on and get staff to use them. We're doing a presentation of the observation we've done and writing a proposal to adopt the tool and the template so we can use that as one of our reporting methods.

It's given us a better insight on what happens on the ward, and we've used the information we gained from the observation to write it up as a hierarchical task analysis — a series of boxes and tasks that have to be done and the order they have to be done in to achieve the overall task of administering medication to a patient. Although it's specific to just one ward, the general principles would be the same everywhere. It's useful to get that knowledge of 'work as done'. It doesn't matter what area you apply it to, it's adaptable and you can look at different things in different environments.

Going forward we think we need to find an incident where an observation might be useful and trial it and support staff in using it.

We don't think you need a training package for it. We think it is something we do anyway: we watch people, we talk to people, and we see what's happening on a normal daily basis. It's part and parcel of being a healthcare professional. You watch patients, you see if they're deteriorating, you observe the unseen clues. It's taking that experience we already have and using it to identify those same trigger points when you're watching somebody do their work. We've got guidelines and the main goal is to observe whatever you're observing but actually it doesn't matter what area you apply it to. It is adaptable so you can change things.

## Conclusions

Observation is a good tool; it is simple to use and you can adapt it to almost anything. You can also spend as much time or as a little time as you want on it.

It can be used to observe something that you do on the ward, to evaluate a process or way of working, or used to decide whether you want to continue something or if something needs an improvement step somewhere. It is useful to use observations as a response to a patient safety incident and to understand how things happened on the day. We concentrated on medication, but equally you could observe a process in the theatre. We observed an entire medication round but if you are short of time, you could just observe it for two or three patients.

Observation is one tool within an armoury of investigative tools that we've got that we should start using. It provides different information to some of the other tools. We think if we had done RCA with a series of statements, which is currently what we do, with maybe some interviews, we wouldn't have found out about the congestion of the corridor, the congestion in the room, the size of the table and the fact that there were factors that interrupted the workflow. If you asked us to write a statement about a drug error, we wouldn't have included the table in the setting, we wouldn't have included the congestion in the room, we wouldn't have included the 19 other distractions prior to the one that made us lose our train of thought.

With observations you immediately get a sense of how the ward or area feels; you get a feel for the leadership just by being there. You can walk into the clinical area and pick up that they're having a bad day just within about five or six steps. You don't get that from the statement and you probably don't get that from an interview, unless somebody tells you that it's a bad day. But when you walk onto a ward, you can feel the atmosphere and you can feel the stress that's on it. Likewise, you can feel if the staff are having a good day. If you walk onto a ward that has got good leadership, it feels very different to a ward that's under pressure. Even if a ward is under pressure, it still feels different with good leadership. You can tell straight away that a ward is well organised and has everything under control. You can't get that from statements; it's something you have to witness yourself.

PSIRF introduces the Human Factors of understanding work as done as opposed to work as imagined. We went along with an idea of what we would see, but we wouldn't have seen the problems the ward had if we hadn't have done the observation. There were things that you wouldn't have thought about if you hadn't seen it. And that's probably the strength of the observation. Observations add Human Factors to the investigation.

> ### Reflections from the Frontline
> 
> - Although observations are a simple and often effective tool, there can be some unintended and potentially critical challenges to completing them effectively.
> - Observations mean following staff as they complete a task. In a hospital setting, this would mean more people on a ward or in an ambulance setting with an observer in a spare seat. This level of access can be difficult, given that services are under ongoing extreme pressure. Managers may feel that they do not want more people around their staff or patients because it is already 'too busy' or there is not the 'capacity' to facilitate a visit. This is a common issue with patient safety work, and a paradox as high levels of demand are when learning is most critical to identify risks to patient safety.
> - Another challenge is deciding who completes the observation. For example, clinical versus non-clinical observers bring strengths and weaknesses to an observation. A clinician brings the experience of having often completed the task themselves or at least empathising with how those being observed feel during the process. A non-clinician may not have a lot of knowledge on the task being observed and could potentially risk not highlighting key points of excellence or potential issues. However, a non-clinician can bring a fresh perspective to an observation; looking through a lens of inexperience brings an independence and the ability to ask why tasks are completed in a certain way that others may simply accept as the norm.
> - An important part of the observation is feeding back on findings. Feedback itself is a learned skill and feeding back on another colleague's work can be a particularly delicate process. If the observer is not allowed the appropriate amount of time to provide feedback or is not trained in effective ways of giving feedback, there is a potential that any learning identified might not be given the attention it needs, or that it may be considered critical and generate defensiveness.
> - If possible, a mix of experiences and views to an observation is beneficial, while also ensuring that senior managers are supportive of the work being carried out. Also allow for the appropriate amount of time to share any learning identified.

## References

Bowling, A. (2014). *Research methods in health* (4th edition). Maidenhead: Open University Press.

Hollnagel, E. and Clay-Williams, R. (2022). *Implementing Science: The Key Concepts* (1st edition). Oxfordshire: Routledge.

McCambridge, J. et al. (2014). 'Systematic review of the Hawthorne effect: new concepts are needed to study research participation effects' in *Journal of Clinical Epidemiology*, 67; pp. 267–77.

McKay, J. et al. (2016). 'Human factors in general practice — early thoughts on the educational focus for specialty training and beyond' in *Education for Primary Care*, 27: pp. 162–71.

Morgan, L. and Bowie, P. (2020). *In-Situ Structured Observation Guide (I-SOG) for exploring human work in healthcare*. Unpublished.

Sedgwick, P., Greenwood N. (2015). 'Understanding the Hawthorne effect' in *British Medical Journal*, p. 351. DOI: 10.1136/bmj.h4672.

Stanton, N.A. et al. (2013). *Human factors methods: a practical guide for engineering and design* (2nd edition). Aldershot: Ashgate Publishing.

## Reading

Bayramzadeh, S. et al. (2018). 'Using an integrative mockup simulation approach for evidence-based evaluation of operating room design prototypes' in *Applied Ergonomics*, 70: pp. 288–99.

Bowie, P. and Jeffcott, S. (2016). 'Human factors and ergonomics for primary care' in *Education for Primary Care*, 27: pp. 86–93.

Braithwaite, J., Wears, R.L. and Hollnagel, E. (2015). 'Resilient health care: turning patient safety on its head' in *International Journal for Quality in Health Care*, 27: pp. 418–20.

Branaghan, R.J. (2018). 'Human factors in medical device design: methods, principles, and guidelines' in *Critical Care Nursing Clinics of North America*, 30: pp. 225–36.

Carayon, P. *et al.* (2014). 'Human factors systems approach to healthcare quality and patient safety' in *Applied Ergonomics*, 45: p. 14.

Catchpole, K. *et al.* (2014). 'A human factors subsystems approach to trauma care' in *JAMA Surgery*, 149: pp. 962–8.

Dekker, S. (2011). *Patient Safety: A Human Factors Approach*. Boca Raton: CRC Press.

Deutsch, E.S. *et al.* (2016). 'Leveraging health care simulation technology for human factors research: closing the gap between lab and bedside' in *Human Factors*, 58: pp. 1082–95.

Hayden, E.M. *et al.* (2018). 'Human factors and simulation in emergency medicine' in *Academic Emergency Medicine*; 25: pp. 221–9.

Hignett, S. *et al.* (2015). 'Human factors and ergonomics and quality improvement science: integrating approaches for safety in healthcare' in *BMJ Quality Safety*, 24: pp. 250–4.

Ratwani, R.M. *et al.* (2018). 'A usability and safety analysis of electronic health records: a multi-center study' in *Journal of the American Medical Informatics Association*, 25: pp. 1197–201.

Valdez, R.S. and Holden, R.J. (2016). 'Health care human factors/ergonomics fieldwork in home and community settings' in *Ergonomics in Design*, 24: pp. 4–9.

Vosper, H. and Hignett, S.A. (2018). 'UK perspective on human factors and patient safety education in pharmacy curricula' in *American Journal of Pharmaceutical Education*, 82: p. 6184.

Vosper, H., Hignett, S. and Bowie, P. (2018). 'Twelve tips for embedding human factors and ergonomics principles in healthcare education' in *Medical Teacher*, 40: pp. 357–63.

**Appendix 1** *In-Situ* Structured Observation Guide (I-SOG) for exploring Human Work in Healthcare. (Morgan and Bowie 2020, unpublished.)

| Date: | Location: | Participant role: |
|---|---|---|

| Work System Element / PIFs | Example Questions & Prompts | Your Notes / Sketches / Photos |
|---|---|---|
| **People** <br> *Personal (physical, cognitive, mental)* <br> *Training and experience* | • Who are the people doing the work? <br> • Explore relevant personal factors <br> • Are roles defined? <br> • Are they trained to complete the task? | |
| **Tasks** <br> *Complexity* <br> *Time pressures* <br> *Workloads* | • What are the main tasks involved in this process? <br> • Is there variation between how people complete the tasks? Which tasks? Why? <br> • Do you need to describe and understand how the task is done? Is the task you are seeing as it has been described? <br> • Can staff describe the work? | |
| **Tools & Technology** <br> *Human-technology interaction and design* <br> *Design of work procedures* | • Do staff consider the technologies/ procedures relevant and usable? <br> • Are they maintained / updated? <br> • Are there obvious use-errors / design issues? <br> • Are there 'supports' i.e. notes to guide use anywhere? | |
| **Physical Environment** <br> *Ambient environment* <br> *Workspace design* | • Explore environment issues: is the lighting adequate, temperature appropriate and noise doesn't inhibit or distract from tasks? <br> • Is this space appropriate for this task? <br> • Where are tasks completed? <br> • Walkthrough a critical task in the space | |
| **Organisational Factors** <br> *Communication* <br> *Social and team* <br> *Leadership, management & supervision* <br> *Handover* <br> *Culture* | • Where is essential information held? <br> • How is new information flagged? <br> • Are there multiple sources of the same information? <br> • Are there issues with resourcing? <br> • What are the processes of work? <br> • Is there variation? <br> • Does this match with what was described? <br> • Explore social and team issues e.g. leadership, handover, supervision, culture | |
| **External Influences** | • What is the national context? <br> • Are there policy, political, regulatory, research agendas influencing work? | |

| Guidance Notes for I-SOG Users Conducting WT3 | General Questions to Consider |
|---|---|
| • Target audience — Healthcare groups interested in understanding and improving Human Work.<br>• Explain your role and purpose of activity.<br>• Multiple data sources (Note: not all PIFs, questions and prompts may be relevant depending on topic):<br>   o Observe a Unit (e.g. hospital ward or individual tasks or activity) and apply verbal walkthrough analysis.<br>   o Gather multiple & diverse perspectives of system users.<br>   o Identify and explore influence of PIFs.<br>   o Review documentation e.g. job aids, checklists/procedures, protocols, policies, incident data, complaints.<br>   o Record observations on the I-SOG, include sketches and/or upload photos (use as a living document).<br>• Note how performance varies (adaptations), how and why.<br>• Triangulate your data sources and interpret aggregated information.<br>• Identify and explore mismatches between work as done and work as imagined.<br>• Conclude with a working summary of work as done and work as imagined. | • What makes anything difficult?<br>• What surprises you?<br>• What do you adapt?<br>• What can go wrong?<br>• What PIFs can lead to harm?<br>• What can be improved and how? |

| Performance Influencing Factor | Explanation/Examples |
|---|---|
| *Personal* | • Personal factors may vary over time and are individual to a person, but may include stress, low morale, boredom, under or over confidence, complacency, poor fitness, poor mental or physical health, age, and/or being under the influence of drugs or alcohol. It also includes being affected by chronic or acute fatigue. |
| *Training and experience* | • Task performance can be adversely affected by a lack of familiarity with a task or inadequate experience of performing a task, poor training or mentoring quality, a lack of training or a time gap between training and doing the task, and/or a lack of opportunity to develop sufficient competence. |
| *Task* | • Task factors are related to excessive demands of the task, excessively high (or low) workload, working under time pressure, complex tasks demanding high levels of concentration, tasks which are very monotonous and repetitive, situations with many distractions, interruptions or divided attention, or non-standard activities. |
| *Human-technology interaction and design* | • The equipment that people interact with, the conditions of that interaction or the workspace can induce failure. There are several examples, including poorly presented information or a lack of information, too much automation (causing low situational awareness), poor quality alarms or alarm overload, poor equipment positioning, poor quality or reliability of equipment, inappropriate work tools for the task, unclear signs and signals, inadequate workplace access or workspace arrangement, or factors that make the task more difficult, such as the use of personal protective equipment. |
| *Design of work procedures* | • Procedures or work instructions can make error more likely through being absent or highly variable in task method, or by being inaccurate, poorly presented, unintelligible, overly complex and/or unclear. |

(*Continued*)

| Performance Influencing Factor | Explanation/Examples |
|---|---|
| Ambient environment | • The ambient environment can present significant challenges to performance and may include the weather, thermal environment, lighting, noise, air quality and/or the presence of health hazards. |
| Workspace design | • Workspace designs that fail to consider human limitations, needs and capabilities can introduce risks that impact on the physical and psychological well-being of the workforce which in turn affects performance and productivity. |
| Communication | • Communication can be verbal, nonverbal, or written (including electronic) and can be adversely affected by a high communications workload, poor phrasing or low communication standards, language differences and heavy accents, the content of the information, the quality and method of communication and the reliability/quality of communications equipment. |
| Social and team | • Social and team factors may include factors affecting teamwork, such as difficult relationships and team dynamics, sub-optimal coordination and communication, and/or a lack of team maturity. It can also include inadequately defined roles and responsibilities, work scheduling, staffing levels and poor shift handover, as well as poor supervision, poor safety culture and a lack of focus on organisational factors during the management of change. |
| External | • External factors that can impact on how human work is done in frontline practice may include national targets, policy and regulatory demands, accreditation standards, global events, and political decision making |

CHAPTER 8

# AcciMaps

*Jayne Wheway and Patrick Waterson*

## Summary

AcciMaps have been used in healthcare for a number of years, although mostly by academics and Human Factors specialists. However, interest is increasing as organisations seek to find a useable and useful systems model for healthcare investigations and learning focused on a single, or more recently, multiple similar patient safety incidents. This needs to be practical and understandable by the clinical and non-clinical healthcare teams.

The original template, designed by Svendung and Rasmussen (2002), was then described in guidance by Branford *et al.* (2009). This approach has been adopted in this chapter with examples to illustrate the construction of an AcciMap. Case studies in practice are detailed later in the chapter to provide evidence and encouragement to try AcciMaps in local organisations and across healthcare systems.

## Background

The AcciMap systems model was created as an accident investigation tool, initially for rescue services in Sweden, and is now used extensively in safety critical industries worldwide. Using a graph template, a visual representation is formed for a particular incident or adverse event scenario (Svedung and Rasmussen, 2002). It represents the causal flow and contributory factors of events at various systemic levels, such as management, regulating bodies and individual processes. This creates a means of analysing the series of events and decision-making processes that were found to have occurred throughout the sociotechnical system resulting in a loss of control and, consequently, the incident/adverse event.

In practical terms within healthcare, an AcciMap can appear complex and chaotic if presented as a finished diagram to those unfamiliar with systems models. However, with explanation of the model and exploration of the incident or event, it can provide an opportunity to highlight the factors that contributed across the system and not only the immediate causes identified at the time (Wheway and Jun, 2021). Vitally, this includes the interactions between the contributory factors at all levels and so encourages an examination across the hierarchy, such as the team, organisation and national bodies alongside the individuals involved at the frontline that resulted in an unwanted outcome.

The use of AcciMaps can enable an investigator or (preferably) an investigation team to build on the information found from incident reports, interviews and other documentation or intelligence, and check this out with subject matter and Human Factors experts. This can helpfully include those involved in the incident and those with leadership and management oversight as gaps are highlighted and the team move towards forming remedial actions to reduce the risk of future harm.

Branford *et al.* (2009) provided the seminal guidance on the approach to the formation of an AcciMap. They describe the coherent 'multi-layered diagram' showing the 'causal remoteness from the outcome' and their interactions, which can then identify problem areas to 'improve the safety of the system and prevent similar occurrences.'

Branford *et al.*'s (2009) steps, adapted by NHS Education for Scotland (unpublished) are summarised as follows:

Step 1. Create a blank AcciMap format.
Step 2. Identify the outcome(s).
Step 3. Identify the contributory factors.
Step 4. Insert the causal links.
Step 5. Fill the gaps.
Step 6. Team check and validate.
Step 7. Make recommendations.

# Steps to Construct an AcciMap

The construction of an AcciMap can be developed by using a large blank sheet of paper with an outline template (as shown in Figure 8.1) and the use of sticky notes during an in-person workshop with relevant colleagues (investigation/patient safety team and/or those involved in the incident and/or relevant subject matter experts, with Human Factors expertise input). Or the AcciMap can be developed electronically using software such as Visio (https://systemsthinkinglab.wordpress.com/accimap/), LucidChart (www.lucidchart.com) or Miro (https://miro.com/index/). The use of collaborative working software, such as Google slides, may provide a useful platform for an online, collaborative workshop.

Alternatively, the investigation or Human Factors lead may develop the first draft of the AcciMap individually from the incident information (of whatever is available) and present to a group, as described above, from which point iterations can be made as the contributory factors are clarified and further information is found.

The steps described below in how to construct an AcciMap will be illustrated by the following examples:

- **Example 1:** An illustrative example concerning an investigation into a single incident was developed (by NHS Education for Scotland). It describes an older person, with early signs of dementia, who has been admitted from her care home to a medical ward due to a fall. She is later prescribed insulin and receives an overdose over several days due to a prescribing error on the ward.
- **Example 2:** A cluster of patient safety incident reports from across England (from the National Reporting and Learning System) in relation to testicular torsion have described delays in every part of the care pathway: referral, assessment, diagnosis, access to senior/specialist advice, commencement of surgery and transfer. This was triangulated with other data such as Royal College position papers and protocols. In using this documentation to create a SEIPS model for the situation at that time, the causal links and stakeholders' underlying assumptions started to emerge.

**Step 1: Create a Blank AcciMap Format on Which to Arrange the Contributory Factors**
Separate the sheet of paper into the relevant number of sections with the headings of the four hierarchical levels on the left-hand side and horizontal lines separating each level.

**AcciMap Analysis of...**

| Government & Regulatory Bodies | |
| Organisational and Management Behaviour | |
| Team and Group Behaviour | |
| Individual Behaviour | |
| Outcomes | |
| Surroundings | |

**AcciMap Analysis of...**

| Government & Regulatory Bodies | |
| National Bodies & Associations | |
| Organisational and Management Behaviour | |

**Figure 8.1** A Blank AcciMap Template, and Inset, Alternative Headings for the Rows/Hierarchy Levels

**Step 2: Identify the Outcome(s)**

Identify negative outcomes to be analysed and place them in the 'outcomes' level of the AcciMap (see Figure 8.2a).

It has become practice for the addition of a row for 'surroundings'; the place to jot things that are important to the scene setting, that may add context.

| AcciMap Analysis of... | |
|---|---|
| Government & Regulatory Bodies | |
| Organisational and Management Behaviour | |
| Team and Group Behaviour | |
| Individual Behaviour | |
| Outcomes | |
| Surroundings | |

**Figure 8.2a** Step 2, Adding the Outcomes and Surroundings

Figure 8.2b shows the outcomes and surroundings for example 1, such as 10x error in insulin prescription and blood glucose noted to be very low, and that the patient had had an intercranial bleed prior to admission, respectively.

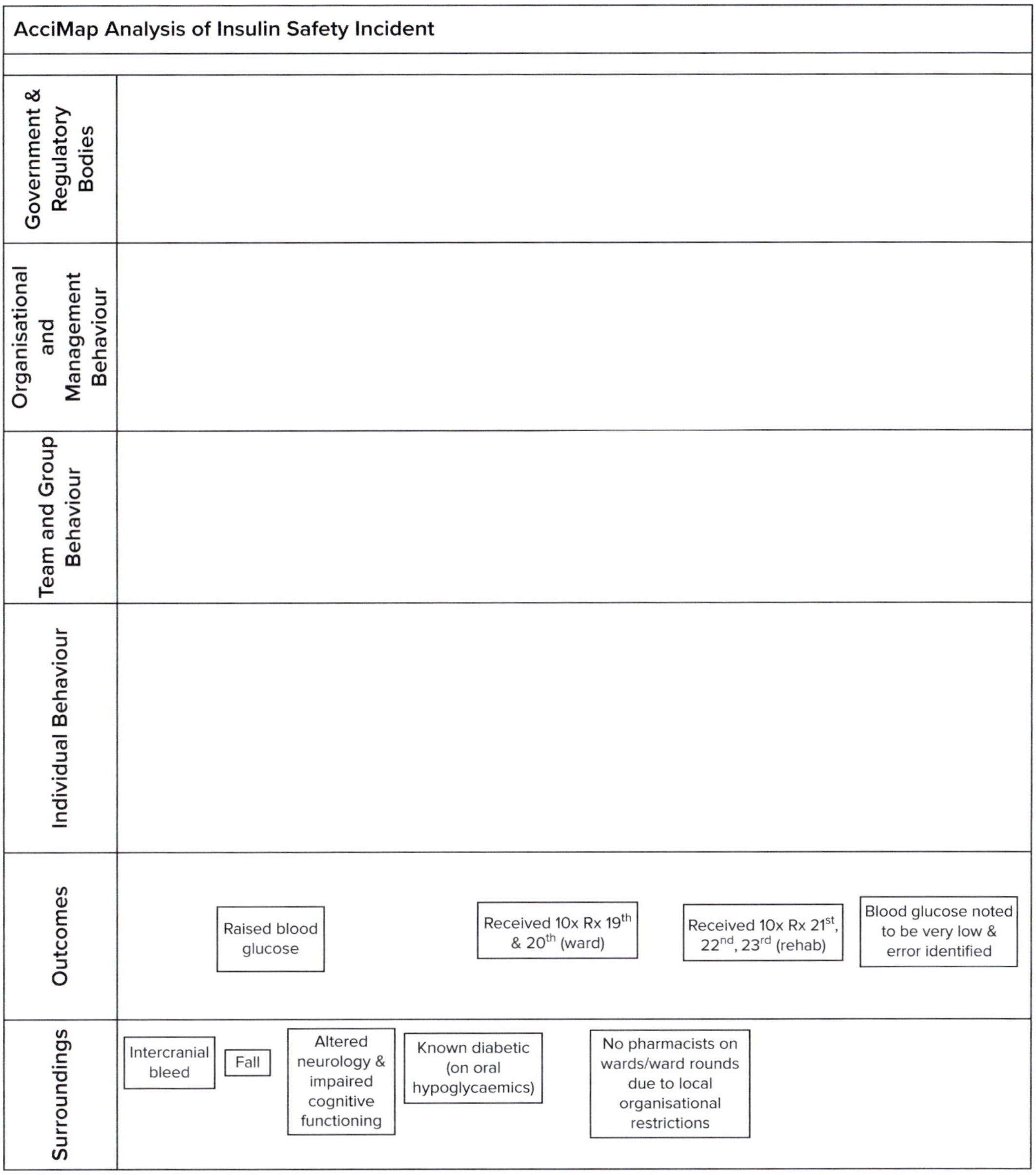

| AcciMap Analysis of Insulin Safety Incident | |
|---|---|
| Government & Regulatory Bodies | |
| Organisational and Management Behaviour | |
| Team and Group Behaviour | |
| Individual Behaviour | |
| Outcomes | Raised blood glucose — Received 10x Rx 19th & 20th (ward) — Received 10x Rx 21st, 22nd, 23rd (rehab) — Blood glucose noted to be very low & error identified |
| Surroundings | Intercranial bleed — Fall — Altered neurology & impaired cognitive functioning — Known diabetic (on oral hypoglycaemics) — No pharmacists on wards/ward rounds due to local organisational restrictions |

**Figure 8.2b** Outcomes and Surroundings for Example 1, Insulin Overdose

Figure 8.2c highlights an outcome that testes necrotised before surgery and had to be removed, and for a surrounding element as the lack of child-friendly facilities at the local hospital.

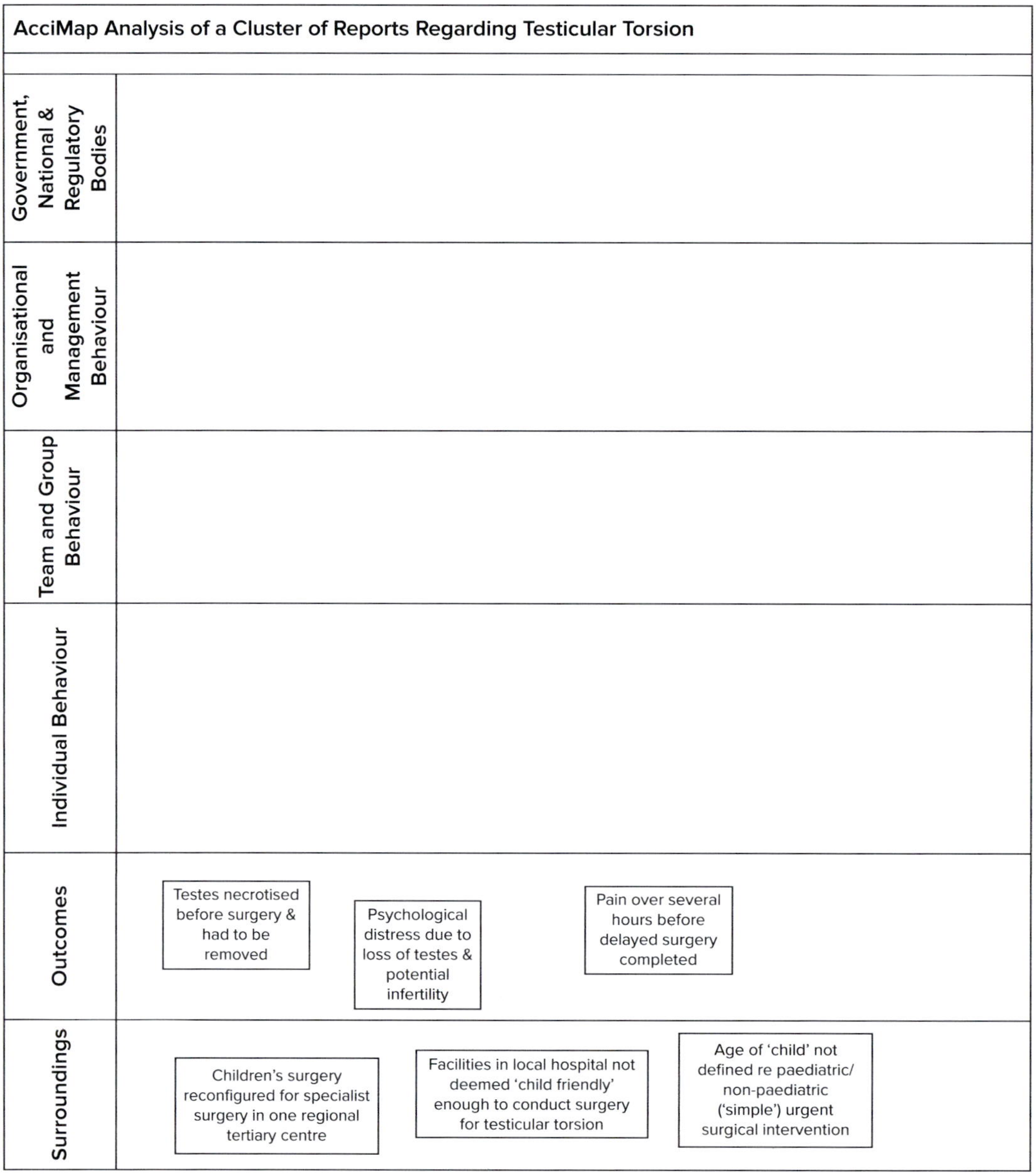

| AcciMap Analysis of a Cluster of Reports Regarding Testicular Torsion | |
|---|---|
| Government, National & Regulatory Bodies | |
| Organisational and Management Behaviour | |
| Team and Group Behaviour | |
| Individual Behaviour | |
| Outcomes | Testes necrotised before surgery & had to be removed • Psychological distress due to loss of testes & potential infertility • Pain over several hours before delayed surgery completed |
| Surroundings | Children's surgery reconfigured for specialist surgery in one regional tertiary centre • Facilities in local hospital not deemed 'child friendly' enough to conduct surgery for testicular torsion • Age of 'child' not defined re paediatric/ non-paediatric ('simple') urgent surgical intervention |

**Figure 8.2c** Outcomes and Surroundings for Example 2, Testicular Torsion

## Step 3: Identify the Contributory Factors and the Appropriate AcciMap Level for Each Factor

Make a list of all the contributory factors in the incident (factors without which it would have probably not occurred) and place it (on a sticky note or a text box) into the level it likely occurred. These can be moved around on further information or discussion. See Figure 8.3a and 8.3b for the contributory factors displayed for examples 1 and 2.

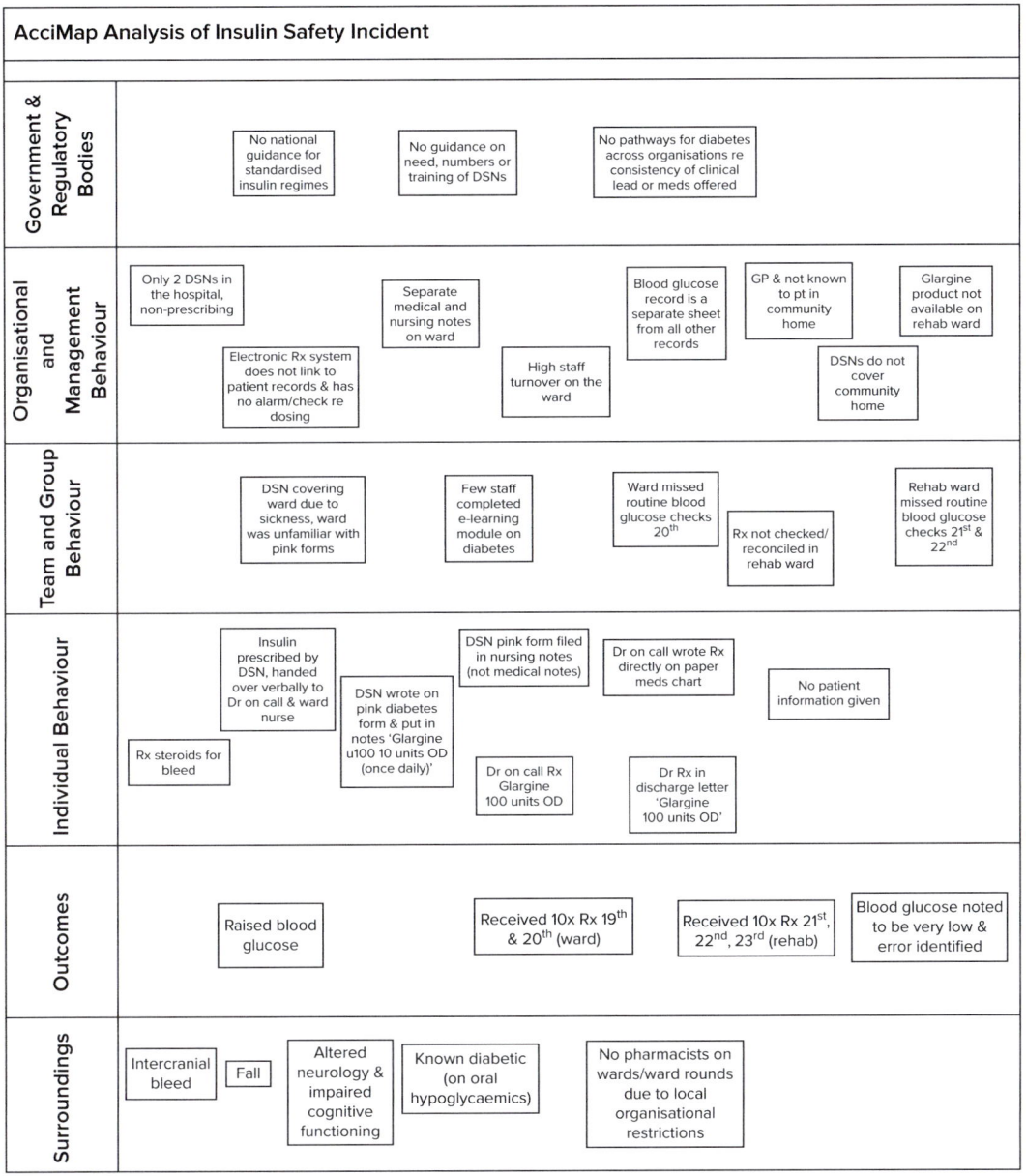

**Figure 8.3a** Contributory Factors Shown for Example 1, Insulin Overdose

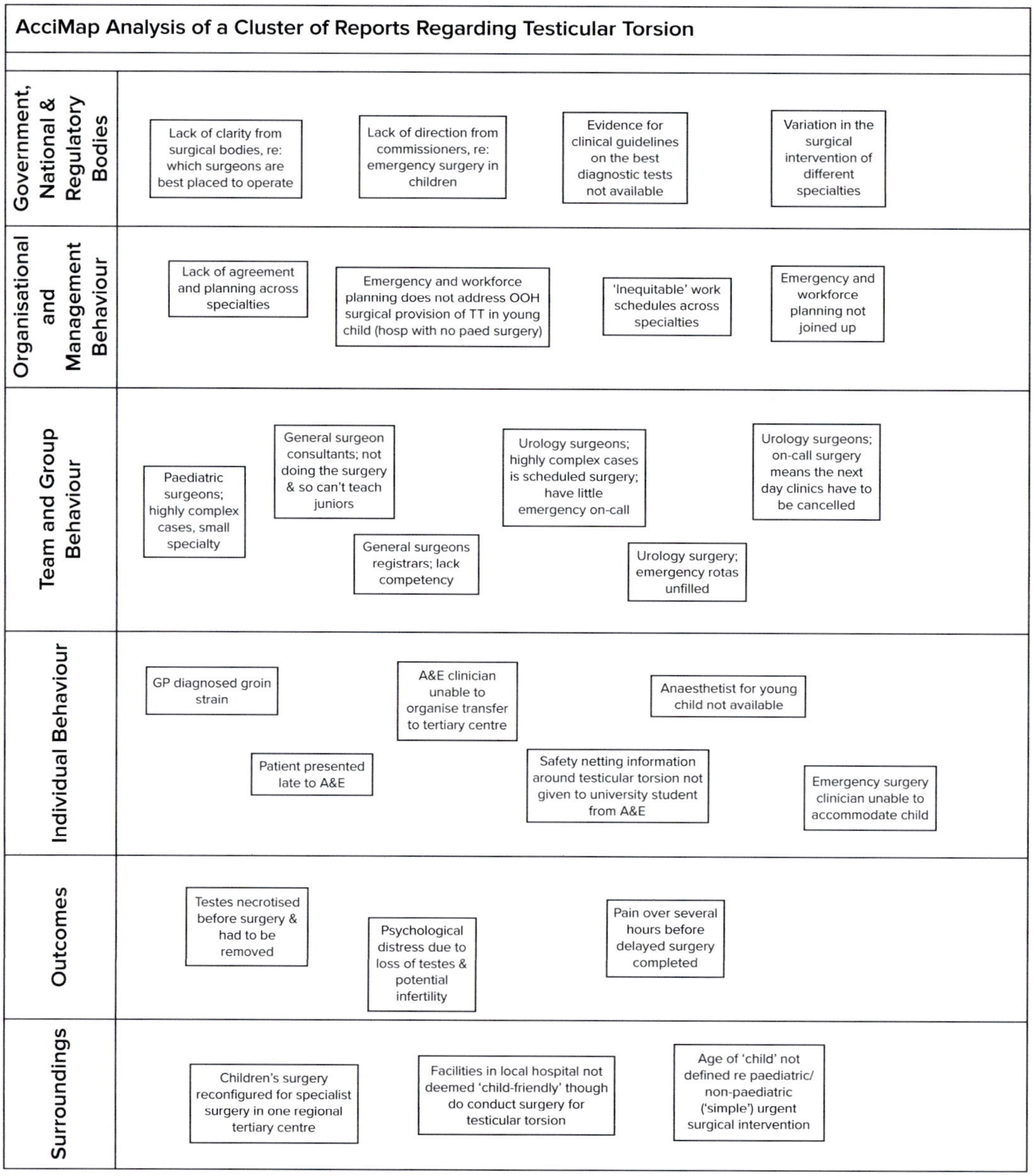

## AcciMap Analysis of a Cluster of Reports Regarding Testicular Torsion

**Government, National & Regulatory Bodies**
- Lack of clarity from surgical bodies, re: which surgeons are best placed to operate
- Lack of direction from commissioners, re: emergency surgery in children
- Evidence for clinical guidelines on the best diagnostic tests not available
- Variation in the surgical intervention of different specialties

**Organisational and Management Behaviour**
- Lack of agreement and planning across specialties
- Emergency and workforce planning does not address OOH surgical provision of TT in young child (hosp with no paed surgery)
- 'Inequitable' work schedules across specialties
- Emergency and workforce planning not joined up

**Team and Group Behaviour**
- Paediatric surgeons; highly complex cases, small specialty
- General surgeon consultants; not doing the surgery & so can't teach juniors
- Urology surgeons; highly complex cases is scheduled surgery; have little emergency on-call
- Urology surgeons; on-call surgery means the next day clinics have to be cancelled
- General surgeons registrars; lack competency
- Urology surgery; emergency rotas unfilled

**Individual Behaviour**
- GP diagnosed groin strain
- A&E clinician unable to organise transfer to tertiary centre
- Anaesthetist for young child not available
- Patient presented late to A&E
- Safety netting information around testicular torsion not given to university student from A&E
- Emergency surgery clinician unable to accommodate child

**Outcomes**
- Testes necrotised before surgery & had to be removed
- Psychological distress due to loss of testes & potential infertility
- Pain over several hours before delayed surgery completed

**Surroundings**
- Children's surgery reconfigured for specialist surgery in one regional tertiary centre
- Facilities in local hospital not deemed 'child-friendly' though do conduct surgery for testicular torsion
- Age of 'child' not defined re paediatric/non-paediatric ('simple') urgent surgical intervention

**Figure 8.3b** Contributory Factors shown for Example 2, Testicular Torsion

## Step 4: Insert Causal Links

Draw the links between various factors. There is no limit to how many links can be drawn from one factor. See Figures 8.4a and 8.4b for the causal links added to examples 1 and 2.

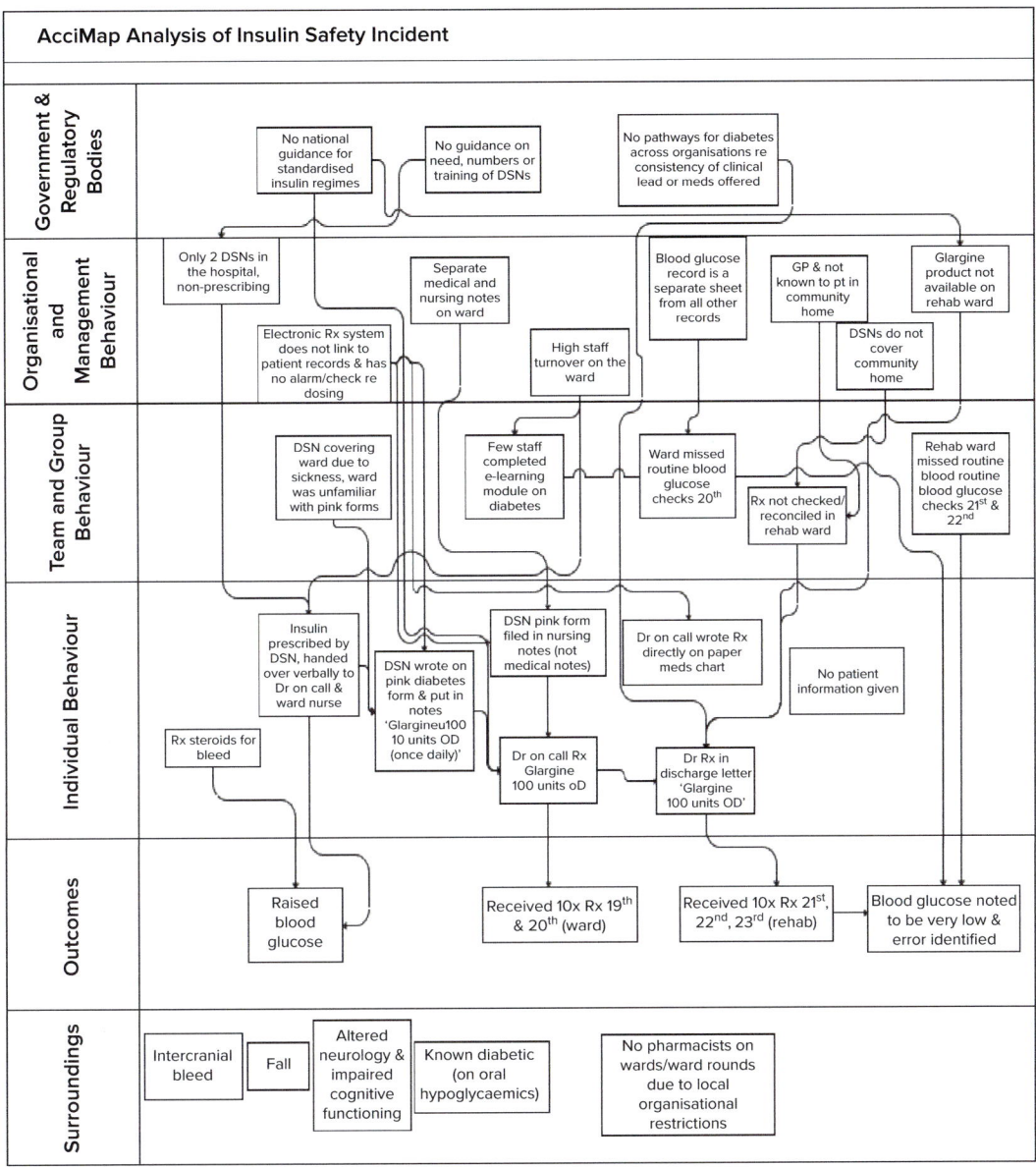

**Figure 8.4a** AcciMap with Causal Links Added to Example 1, Insulin Overdose

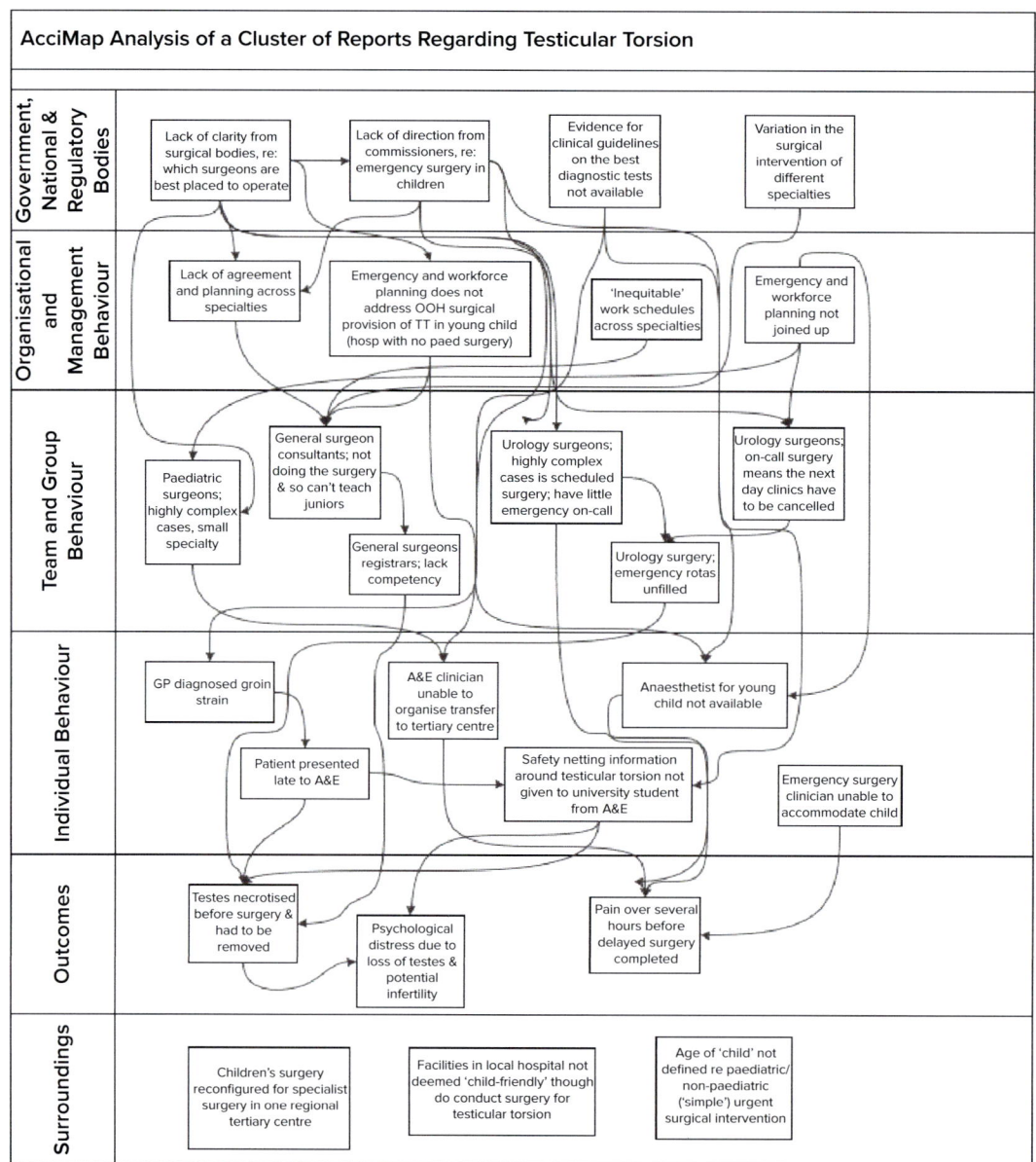

**Figure 8.4b** All Causal Links Added to Example 2, Testicular Torsion

## Step 5: Fill in the Gaps (if any)

Check for gaps/missing contributory factors. Look at all levels and factors to consider if there are more factors, particularly further up the hierarchy; for example, national policy, clinical guidelines, commissioning or procurement decisions. Branford *et al.* (2009) encourages an examination of every factor to consider why it occurred and to extend each factor to at least the level of the organisation.

## Step 6: Team Check and Validate

Gather together people involved/those who are knowledgeable around investigations and/or the clinical area or issue involved to confirm the information on the AcciMap.

This step has been adapted from Branford *et al.*'s (2009) original list, as it is this team working practice that is important in healthcare incident investigation that aims to uncover what happened, why it made sense at the time, how the contributory factors across and within the complex system are interacting, and what remedial actions might improve safety. This team check may be iterative as the process of clarification, considered action and risk management of the proposed changes are completed. It can also add to the shared understanding and reduction of feelings of blame to those who were nearest the incident and to provide a place for interactive exploration for those with the role to create change.

As the AcciMap is near completion it may be useful to use themes for collating groups of factors for understanding or forming actions for change. For instance, in example 1 changes at an organisational level or ward level actions that can be taken immediately (Figure 8.5).

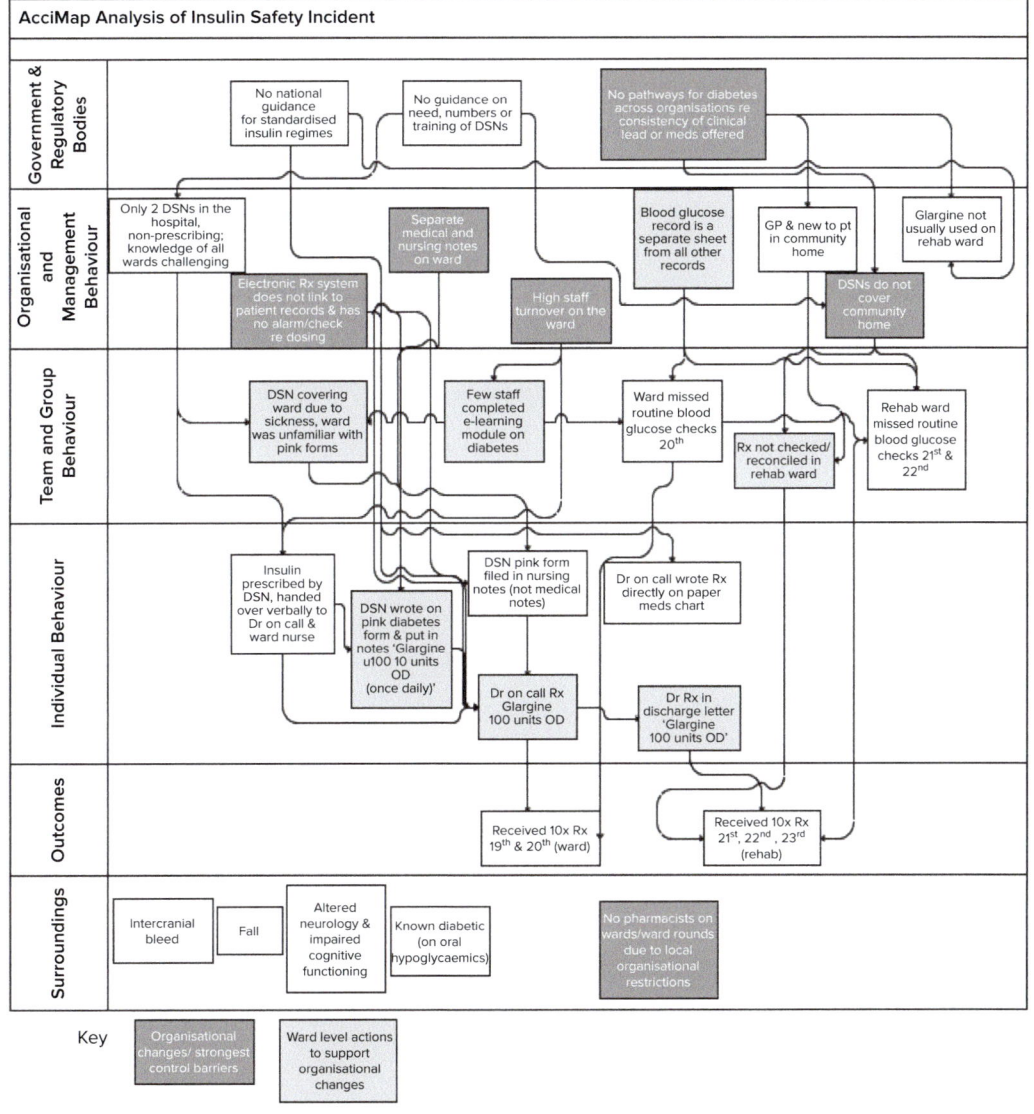

**Figure 8.5** Completed AcciMap with Highlighted Themes for Example 1, Insulin Overdose

**124** Patient Safety: Emerging Applications of Safety Science

### Step 7: Make Recommendations

This follows on closely from the team check as it should fall out of those clarifications and discussions. There may also be value in speaking to others as relevant recommendations are considered; for example, a clinical team in a related area/organisation, such as primary care or children's services, or the quality improvement team working on an issue that could incorporate a recommendation in their work, such as early warning systems or electronic patient prescribing.

Recommendations need to identify specific actions to mitigate contributory factors based on SMART principles – they should be Specific, Measurable, Achievable, Relevant and Time-framed.

## ActorMaps

An ActorMap can be useful to show the individuals, teams and organisations involved in the AcciMap or may be relevant to the incident by way of decisions, risk management or work planning. Figure 8.6 shows an ActorMap for example 1.

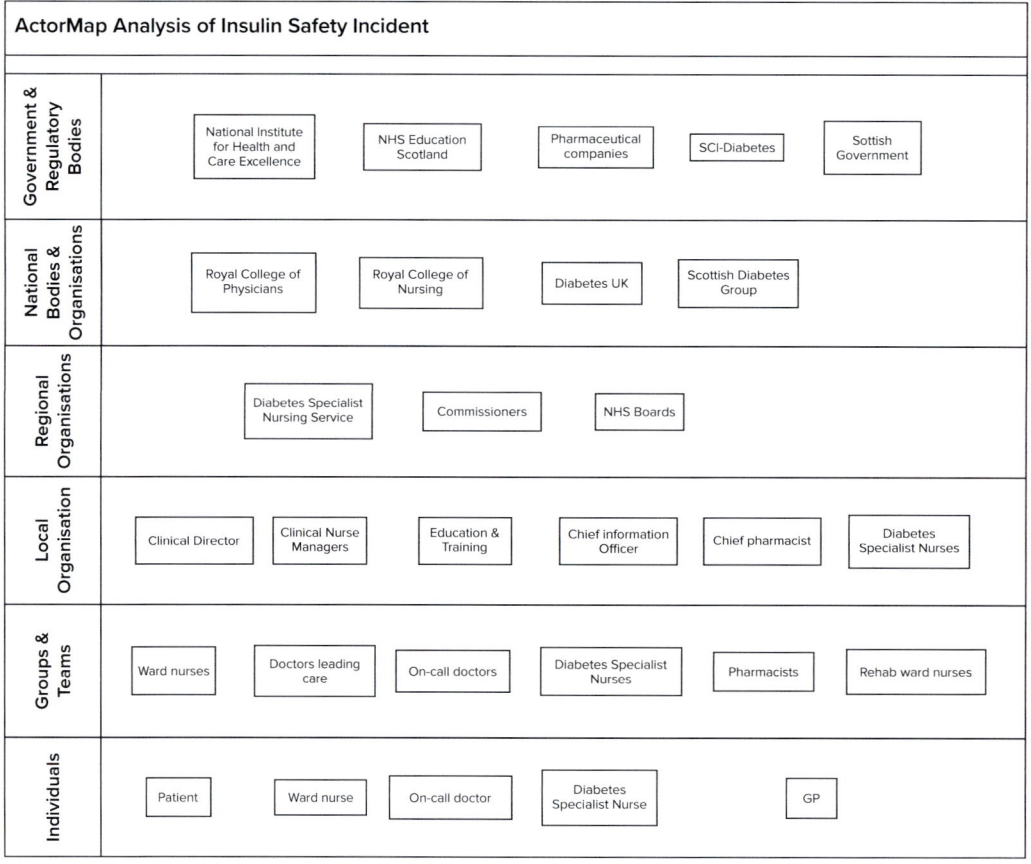

**Figure 8.6** ActorMap Analysis of the Insulin Safety Incident

# Final Thoughts

In comparison with other system models, especially those used for accident investigation, AcciMaps are simple and the theory is little more than that of systems thinking and systems theory. However, a systems approach is not yet embedded in healthcare. It is still commonplace to find that patient safety incident reporting concludes that the staff member involved has been sent for 'training' and 'competencies support' with no mention of any other contributory factors or surrounding contextual information, so nothing more than the outcome and the individual actions (not even the individual decisions included) would have been entered on the AcciMap.

In the short term, there is still a significant amount of training and education required to embed and value the Human Factors investigation approaches, such as the use of AcciMap as essential and not an 'added extra', to pause to gather relevant people (in the clinical area, the non-clinical work area as relevant, the managers/leaders, patient safety, quality improvement and Human Factors professionals) to explore the incident or cluster of incidents or events in order to focus on the contributory factors and reflect on the remedial actions that may increase patient and staff safety.

Patients, families and carers are also increasingly expressing a desire to be involved in more than the final outcome of the investigation and this may be a useful tool if consideration is given in how this might be best achieved. The introduction of the Patient Safety Partners (patients, service users, carers or other lay people) to all NHS organisations in England may be a useful contribution to this agenda.

Some patient safety experts prefer AcciMap to the SEIPS model, but the same research showed that others prefer SEIPS (Wheway and Jun, 2021). SEIPS is currently being heralded as an example of a flexible transferable model for patient safety in healthcare, which it is, but AcciMap has the advantage of highlighting hierarchy. More research on the use of AcciMaps and other systems models would provide a suite of tools that may usefully support not only patient safety investigation but also systems thinking across healthcare.

# Acknowledgements

The authors would like to acknowledge Paul Bowie and Thomas Jun for their work on the NHS Education Scotland insulin example used in this chapter and Paul for allowing us to use his figures.

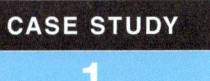

**CASE STUDY 1** — Wendy Halliburton, Patient Safety Lead, Academic Health Science Network North East & North Cumbria (AHSN NENC)

## Background

Working as the Patient Safety Specialist in an Acute & Community provider, I was interested in exploring techniques for improving incident investigation and identifying a wider range of causal factors to support the development of achievable and effective recommendations. At the time, PSIRF was being piloted and while it required that incident investigations utilise a systems approach, there was no recommended tools or available training. I looked to identify and evaluate systemic accident analysis (SAA) tools that would be suitable to be taught to and applied by Patient Safety Incident investigators undertaking investigations within an acute trust, the majority of whom are clinicians by background and not Human Factors specialists.

Following review, the four most utilised SAA tools were identified as AcciMap (Rasmussen, 1997; Rasmussen and Svedung, 2000), Systems-Theoretic Accident Model and Processes (STAMP) (Leveson, 2004), Functional Resonance Analysis Method (FRAM) (Hollnagel, 2004) and Human Factors Analysis and Classification System (HFACS) (Wiegmann and Shappell, 2001, 2003). HFACS is an epidemiological model; however, the difference between this and a systemic approach is subtle (Underwood and Waterson, 2014).

The review identified that AcciMap was easier to understand with an 'output' diagram which effectively explained the sequence of events, communicated findings and identified recommendations. It also required less time for analysis, although some practitioners found the arrows confusing (Salmon et al., 2012; Underwood and Waterson, 2014; Kee, 2017; Igene et al., 2017; Woodier, 2017; Goncalves Filho et al., 2019; Igene and Johnson, 2020; Wheway, 2020). In contrast, Woodier (2017) found practitioners preferred HFACS, as its prescriptive nature made it easier to learn and apply. Tools with a taxonomy, such as HFACS and STAMP, were useful for aggregated analysis, and specific healthcare-based taxonomies had been developed for HFACS (Murray et al., 2017; Salmon et al., 2012; Woodier, 2017).

The study was designed to gain insight into whether SAA tools could be used by practitioners for PSIIs, and whether the tools achieved their function, were easy to learn and use and were applicable to future incident investigations.

## What We Did

The study took place in a combined acute and community NHS Trust. All staff who had led serious incident (SI) investigations over the previous two years, and all senior patient safety staff who facilitated investigations, were invited to participate in the study. Participants were allocated between two groups to ensure a mixture of lead investigators, patient safety leads and patient safety coordinators.

The two groups received training on each method in reverse sequence to adjust for order bias in the evaluation (Wheway, 2020; Woodier, 2017). The sessions were delivered face-to-face and via video link simultaneously; they were also recorded for some staff to access at their convenience.

The training sessions included a short introductory session on systems thinking and SAA tools (15 minutes), followed by a 45-minute face-to-face training session for each method. The sessions gave background to each method and presented a standardised approach to application. Each session also included a worked example. After each session, participants were provided with a handbook containing the standard guidelines and an additional worked example from Salmon et al. (2012).

Following each taught session, participants completed an analysis using a single case study. On completion they submitted their analysis to the researcher for use (anonymously) in the focus group. The case study was taken from the report 'Placement of nasogastric tubes' (HSIB, 2020). The national investigations by HSIB were considered the 'gold standard' of healthcare incident reports available at the time and had been undertaken using a systems approach (SEIPS) (Carayon et al., 2006) and AcciMap.

Previous studies had evaluated SAA models based on utility and usability. For consistency, and to allow comparison with previous studies, permission was obtained from the authors of the studies to adapt their questionnaires for this study (Underwood et al., 2016; Woodier, 2017). Additional questions were included about future application of the tools. After completion of all training sessions and receipt of the evaluation questionnaires, participants were invited to attend a focus group to further explore the utility, usability and future application of the tools.

In total, 38 staff were invited to participate in the study (Figure 8.7).

## Lessons Learned

There were limitations to the study. Those who participated were a self-selected sample who may have had more opportunity to attend or greater interest in learning about the tools. There was a high 'non-contact' and dropout rate (which may be due to the study taking place during the Covid-19 pandemic). This may have contributed to the consistently positive evaluation of both tools. It was considered that the previous external training session on AcciMap in 2019 may impact on the responses; however, a similar proportion of participants stated they were familiar with HFACS. The small sample size, within a single Trust, will limit the generalisability of the results to a wider population.

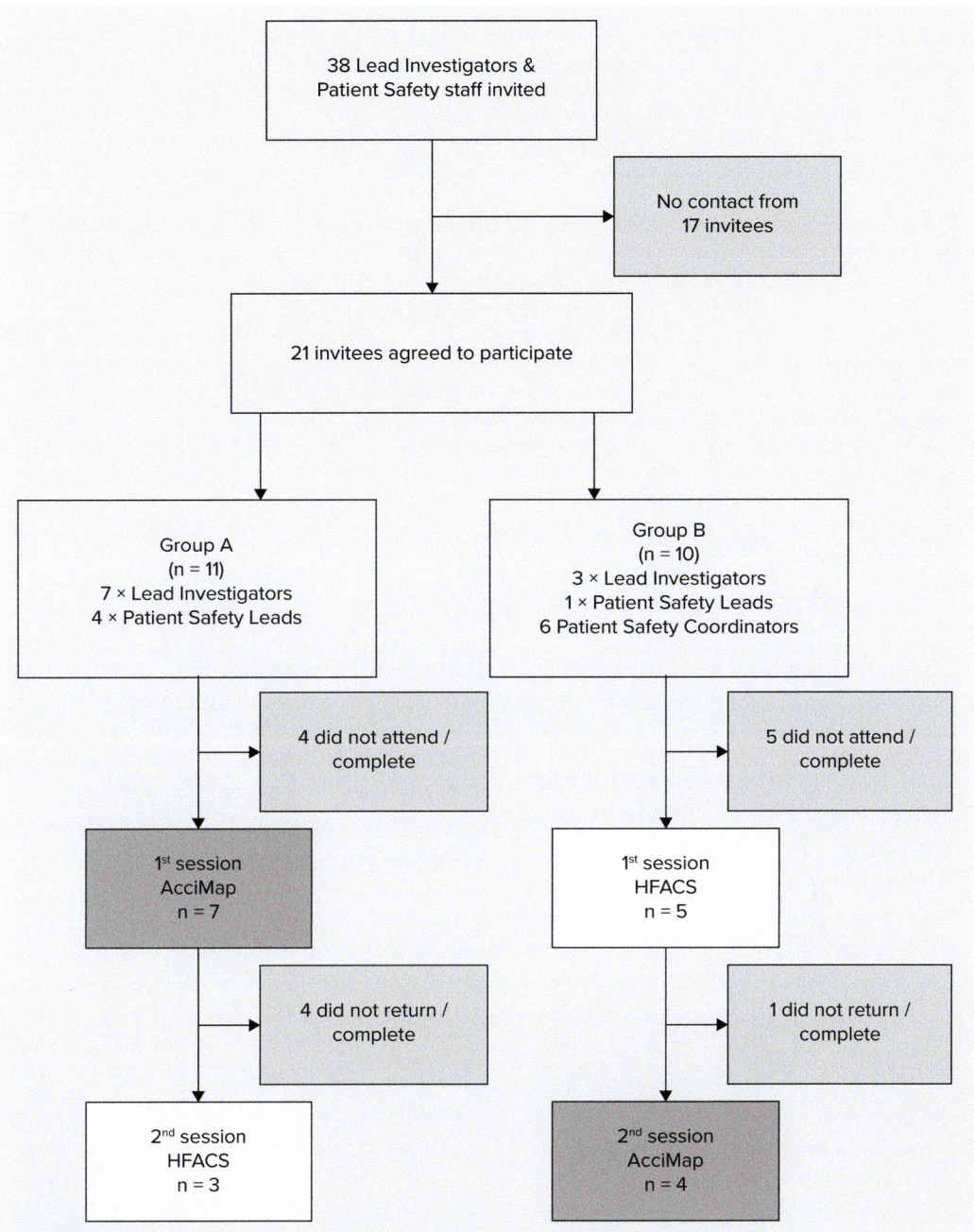

**Figure 8.7** Flow Diagram of the Participant Involvement in the Study

Respondents may have been guarded in their responses as a single researcher delivered the training, led the focus group and evaluated the responses. Although the questionnaires were anonymous, with a small group of participants who were colleagues of the researcher, they may have considered they could be identified through their responses.

## Evaluation and Impact

### Utility

Practitioners agreed that both tools were suitable for analysing incidents. Practitioners identified most of the same factors although they were not always assigned to the same level (AcciMap), tier or code (HFACS). Other researchers have found that while the phrasing and placement may differ, the factors identified were the same and practitioners identified similar recommendations (Igene et al., 2017).

A high proportion of respondents agreed the tools identified technical components; individual and/or team elements, decisions or actions; organisational issues; environmental issues; and external issues. Most respondents agreed that both methods provided a comprehensive description of the incident and that the methods effectively represented the relationships between system components.

All respondents agreed or strongly agreed that AcciMap correctly identified the causes of an incident, although not all agreed that HFACS achieved this. In contrast, Woodier (2017) found that practitioners liked HFACS because the structure prompted them to identify all the relevant factors, whereas AcciMap had the potential to overlook things.

All participants agreed to some degree that AcciMap was effective at identifying areas for change (recommendations). In the focus group, respondents commented that as the methods helped to identify causal factors that they may have overlooked and also contributory factors that may not be accessible to actions by the Trust, this helped them to focus their efforts on developing actions that were achievable and effective.

> *What it showed is, there is some things in an investigation that you may pick up as being as problem, but if you can't do anything about it [...] we're never going to achieve them.*

> *It did bring out some different things that although we'd covered most avenues there was some things that were highlighted [...] that we could have done.*

> *I found that I had lots of repetition across all of the areas. I am therefore unsure if I was confident that I was using the correct 'evidence' in each of the areas.*

> *It was useful to identify what was way out of our control, such as the external factors, [...] that we can't do anything about, so national guidance, changes in national guidance, and things like that.*

### Usability

Most respondents felt the tools were easy to understand, in particular AcciMap which was described as very user friendly. The majority also thought the tools made it easy to identify contributory factors, unsafe acts or decisions, errors and violations and inadequate controls within the system. Some respondents wanted more clarification with HFACS and suggested a pro forma to populate with the findings; others were more positive about the terms and concepts in HFACS, reflecting the inclusion of a taxonomy.

Within the focus group practitioners expressed a clear preference, with some preferring the structure and prescriptive nature of HFACS and others preferring the freedom of AcciMap. Practitioners felt that the preference for one tool or the other was personal choice or based on the incident type or investigation style. Woodier (2017) found that practitioner preference was based on cognitive styles.

Whilst participants were asked to complete their analysis individually, many chose to work in groups. It was notable that practitioners were more confident to apply HFACS on their own but preferred a team-based approach for AcciMap to allow discussion, develop ideas and establish a consensus. Kee (2017) noted that it is difficult for the novice to know where to put things in AcciMap because there is no 'right' answer.

The participants agreed that the tools were easy to use as a team and promoted a collaborative approach; they proposed working with the MDT for different perspectives and to generate more ideas. Underwood and Waterson (2014) found that discussion between investigators resulted in a consensus that minimised any bias from individual background or experience.

> *We were going to do it on our own and see if we came up with different... outcomes, but we thought it was better to just try to do it together and we found it quite beneficial.*

> *I did it all on my own.*

> *We did it as a team.*

> *[We] did it together, and we found it really useful.*

> *I think if I was doing the HFACS as a starter, I was ok sort of working through that on my own.*

> *I just think doing it as a team and with different, erm, like [PSL1] says, we're nurses but with involvement with clinicians and others, other erm, staff, you know it might have been a little bit better, should we say?*

> *I feel it would be most beneficial within a team review of an incident as this would allow for discussion and agreement by the team.*

> *I feel as though I would have benefitted from having my colleagues there, I suppose to, to do it together, you know, we might have come up with some different ideas.*

> *We have recently used it...as a team, on some incidents that we've done and for us it did bring out some different things that although we thought we'd covered most avenues there was some things that were highlighted...that we could have done.*

> *I do think that if we were to implement that it needs to be done as a team and not one person's opinion...and also different perspectives, as in different teams... because, say, medical engineering come up with different questions...to pharmacy, to nurses, to medics,...so that was evident when we've looked at it on one of our 'real' incidents.*

> *It was the AcciMap one where I think you'd have needed that, probably to bounce off people and say 'well that fits there' and 'what are we going to put in there?', and when you were talking about moving them around, your post its, ...I think that sort of needs discussion with people to say 'where do you, ...where do you put them?*

> *So you're right as in, it would be discussion on which one to use, erm, and then an evaluation after the first time you use it, are your teams happy with it, that you're working with, does it make sense to them?*

Practitioners in this study were divided on the 'output' diagram of AcciMap. In the questionnaire the majority agreed that it was a useful communication tool, but in the focus group, one practitioner found the use of sticky notes confusing and another was concerned that they did not have the IT skills to produce anAcciMap 'graph thing'. Other studies found similar comments, with some declaring AcciMap as chaotic and messy (Woodier, 2017), and others disliking the arrows (Wheway, 2020); whilst others found the diagram helped them to understand the causal relationships (Igene and Johnson, 2020). Practitioners found that the taxonomy in HFACS was useful for classifying the causes of the incident.

### Future application

All respondents agreed that it would be easy for them to become skilled using the methods but most agreed that they would need additional training or expert help to apply the methods. Most respondents felt both methods were appropriate for application to PSIIs.

Respondents were keen to use the AcciMap in their next investigation, although there was recognition that, for both tools, the teams would need further support to apply to a 'live' incident.

> *I do think the first few times we do, if we do decide to use it, we would probably, ...I think our team anyway, would probably need some help, erm, to get things started, and make sure we are on the right track and not go off on a tangent.*

> *I am going to use it on my next [serious incident] to try it out.*

> *Current patient safety team will need help to get out of old habits if this system was agreed.*

> *It would be, discussion on which one to use, erm, and then an evaluation after the first time you use it, are your teams happy with that you're working with, does it make sense to them?.*

> *I feel it would be beneficial to utilize the process in my next incident investigation.*

> *May not be suitable for all investigations I feel it is a tool that would easily be incorporated into the investigation process.*

## Conclusions

Healthcare, like other industries, is complex, and simple linear cause and effect models are inadequate to explain how events occur (Underwood and Waterson, 2014; Underwood et al., 2016; Waterson et al., 2017). The aim of the study I undertook was to identify and evaluate SAA tools that would be appropriate for application to PSIIs within an acute Trust. Patient safety practitioners in healthcare are mostly clinicians by background, and while they have a passion for patient safety, they have had limited Human Factors training or systems knowledge to date. They are keen to adopt tools and methods that will enhance their investigations and support system learning and continuous improvement, but the models need to be accessible, useful and usable (Underwood and Waterson, 2014).

Although the creation of Patient Safety Specialists from within the current workforce means there has been no additional expertise injected into the NHS (NHS England and Improvement, 2020), this study has shown that experienced healthcare investigators can gain the knowledge and confidence to apply SAA tools following an introductory training session.

This is an opportunity to upskill a workforce of passionate healthcare professionals into patient safety specialists, rather than degrading the SAA tools to a simple template to be completed. The value of the SAA tools in healthcare is not their ability to reproduce valid and reliable results time after time, nor in generating a case study worthy of publication, but in the process of investigation.

The practitioners gained the most, not from developing a perfect AcciMap diagram, but from undertaking the analysis as a team, generating discussion, and identifying additional causal factors and effective, achievable areas for change.

If patient safety specialists are to use a systems approach to investigation, they need awareness of and accessibility to the tools, and training on how and when to apply them. Practitioners should be encouraged to embrace SAA tools for their ability to generate ideas and identify relevant causes that are accessible to change and improvement (Waterson *et al.*, 2017). Afterall, learning and improvement is what will make us a safer tomorrow.

---

### CASE STUDY 2

Chris Elston, Patient Safety Education Lead, Acute Trust

## Background

In our acute trust, we wanted to improve the investigation training that we provide for our staff. We wanted to use a Human Factors perspective to look at the contributory factors and causal links behind patient safety incidents and needed a new framework to use.

As our training programme needs to fit around people's normal work, the system had to be undaunting and require little training to use. As our faculty had already received training in the use of the AcciMap tool (Rasmussen, 1997), we decided to add this framework into our 'Introduction to Patient Safety Incident Investigation' training course.

It allowed the use of a framework to base an investigation on as we move towards PSIRF.

A scenario was produced for the training course that was based on several different adverse event reports combined into one incident. The aim was to showcase the value of using the framework and for staff attending the training to be aware of the myriad of contributory factors that lie behind many incidents.

We wanted to get staff thinking about systems and to look for additional contributory factors connected to the event.

## What We Did

The scenario (Box 8.1 shows example scenarios) is sent out to the candidates about two weeks before the course starts and forms the basis of the course over its two sessions. The main protagonists in the incident are interviewed, and the information gleaned from the interviews and the incident report is then used to formulate the AcciMap. Staff were asked to complete an AcciMap around the incident.

### BOX 8.1  Example Scenarios

- Patient is hard of hearing and requires British Sign Language interpreter, leads to misidentification.
- Surgeon is running late due to bed meeting.
- Operating theatre set up for the wrong side operation.
- Does not participate in checklist.
- New member to the team.
- Distractions – answering bleeps.
- Incivility.
- Surgery on wrong knee.
- Incomplete documentation.
- Duty of candour not completed.

We use the following headings in our AcciMap:

**Outcome** — this usually starts out with the incident that caused the investigation but can be added to as the investigation develops. For example, we have had one team decide that an outcome included the impact that the event had on the team with regards to their ability to speak up.
**Physical/individual factors** — what factors are attributable to the people involved in the incident, so the surgeon, the nurse, the patient, reception staff. Civility, being late and a laissez-faire attitude are often identified at this point.
**Technical/operational management** — the factors that are due to the workplace/clinical environment. For our incident this includes the waiting room and the operating theatre. Induction training, culture and the incorrect set-up of theatre are frequent factors here.
**Organisation/hospital management** — in this section we often find meetings, parking, policies and guidelines are identified, alongside culture.
**External factors and Government** — it is here that pressure to reduce the backlog and Covid-19 are often quoted.

We have used a number of different techniques to capture the factors that are identified by the teams. These have included a digital approach using some free applications, such as Google Jamboard, and a more traditional approach of paper and sticky notes or pens. The best approach has been using a system that allows the factor to be moved around the chart, as members of the team will have different opinions of where the factor should sit, and then a discussion will ensue which may result in the factor being moved.

To identify the interactions, it is easier to work up the chart and group related items together. For example, all the training elements, such as induction, 'ask don't tell' and training records would be grouped together and could lead to an area for further investigation.

Capturing the information is proving a little difficult in the scenario we use, so we have been photographing the AcciMap. There will need to be further thought about how the information can be transferred into a report. This could be as simple as keeping the current report format and include the photograph of the completed AcciMap.

The lack of knowledge and experience of the members on the course is not proving to be a barrier for the use of the AcciMap, which supports our assumption that this would be a good tool to introduce our staff to a system framework to base the investigations around.

We have produced a handbook for staff to use as an aide memoire and this includes the AcciMap and an example of when it is used for a favourable outcome.

## Lessons Learned

Every time we use the scenario and get the candidates to complete the AcciMap, there is always new information or a new way to look at the information. This is due to the way the training puts a team together — for example, a biomedical scientist will see other factors that a nurse may not, due to their occupational experience.

This is a strength of the AcciMap as it can be used by everyone; people who are not familiar with the practice that is being examined will see patterns and interactions that those more familiar with the practice do not see. One recommendation that I would make is to have someone unfamiliar with the work area in the investigation team as that will provide richer data.

We often see that without well-described terms of reference for the investigation then there is a possibility that the investigation can either dwell and concentrate on one specific area of an incident or encompass more and more areas.

There is a risk that the AcciMap becomes a list of contributory factors and the interactions are not explored. Without the exploration of these interactions then it is not always possible to see the areas where improvements can be made to strengthen the system. There needs to be some investigation experience to ensure that both of these criticisms are controlled.

The main strength of the AcciMap is that it is simple to use, reasonably self-explanatory and allows multiple perspectives. It can be used when something has gone wrong but equally it can also highlight positive events and discover why they go well. This allows for the learning to be identified and shared all on the same framework.

## Evaluation and Impact

Our next step is to move from training and actually use the AcciMap in the investigation of a patient safety incident. We have been referring to it in all of our patient safety presentations.

There is little difference in the application of the AcciMap between staff groups. All those that have attended the training have been able to identify the multiple contributory factors. This includes staff that are not normally patient facing. Anecdotally, some of the non-patient-facing staff see the interactions easier than the patient-facing staff; for example the biomedical scientists move to making connections quicker than the clinical staff.

Staff feedback shows that the AcciMap training has been well received, with staff finding it easy to use, and also that working in a team provides richer data. This is, in part, due to the different perspectives of the team members. It provides a reminder to look up and out instead of focusing on the proximal situation.

> 'Very useful to go over the scenario ourselves. Many people thought of things others didn't and it really brought a good discussion amongst our group and we were able to see it from different perspectives.'

> 'For those who will be expected to engage with this process it was a good insight of what's to come — I understand that the new process essentially has widened the scope of our current investigation process enabling a better understanding (with the hope of a fairer understanding) of all contributory factors.'

> 'Logical methodology.'

> 'This tool is brilliant. Being able to work upwards from Outcomes to External for identifying causes and then work downwards from External to Outcomes to come up with suggestions for solutions made it a lot easier to go into that zoomed view and not get fixated on just the individual causes.'

Currently we capture the information by photographing the AcciMaps that are produced in the course. One of the challenges we now face is how to transfer this to a report and suggestions for areas to improve. On the course, we use the AcciMap to identify frailties in the system and then invite the candidates to write an action that could strengthen the system. We envisage that this will be the way forward to provide the information in a useful format.

Figures 8.8–8.10 show examples of the AcciMaps drawn up on the course and Figure 8.11 shows the early action plan drawn up.

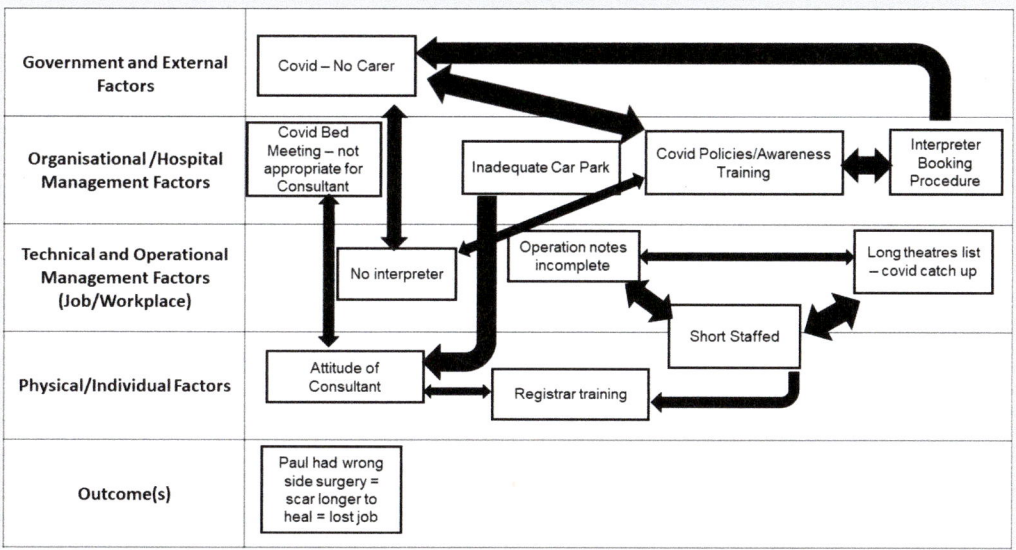

**Figure 8.8** AcciMap Showing the Early Attempts to Identify Interactions

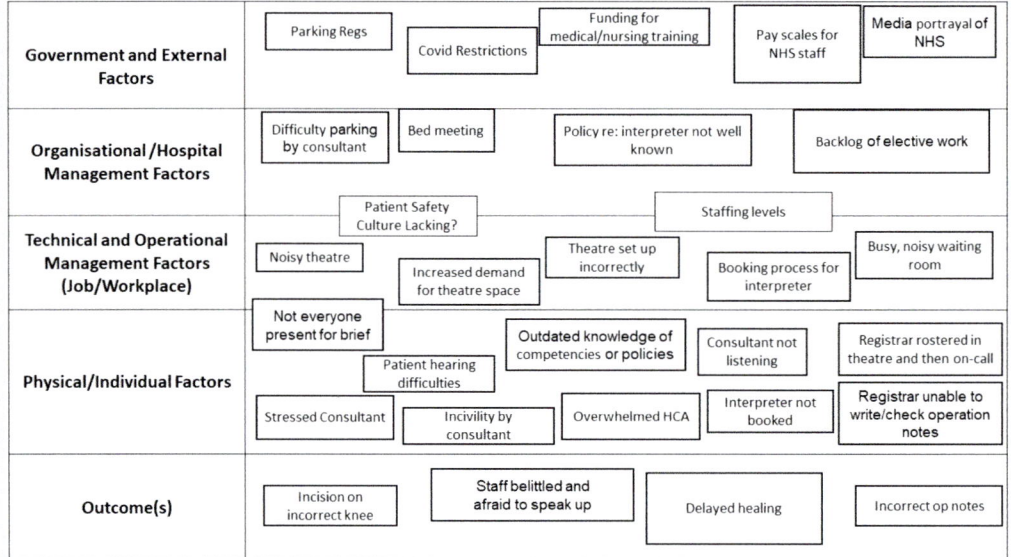

**Figure 8.9** An AcciMap Showing Richness of Data and Beginnings of Action Plan

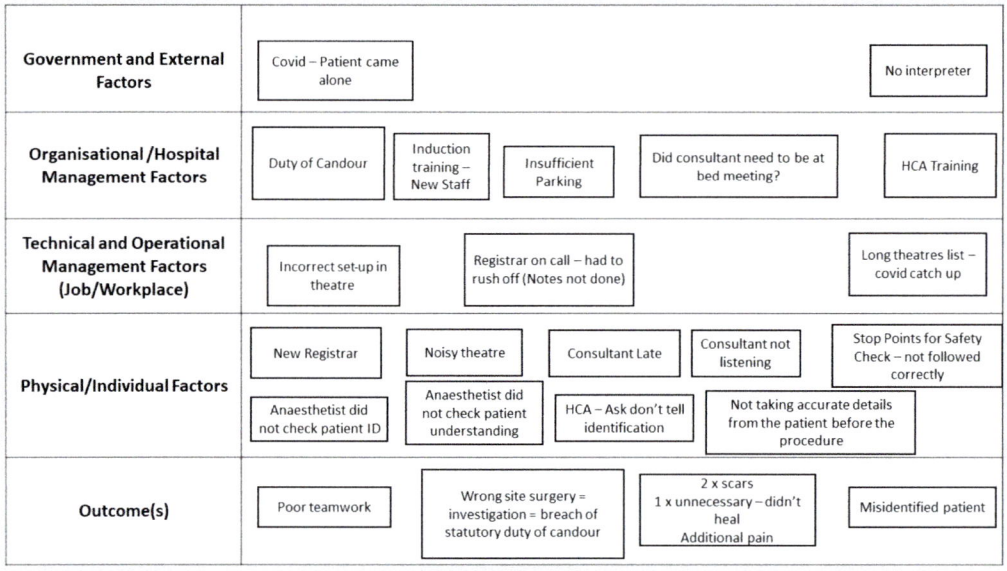

**Figure 8.10** An Example of the Type of Data that can be Delivered Using an AcciMap

### Action Plan
- Review backlog strategy
- De-conflict rostering overlaps
- Review of bed meeting
    - Attendance list
    - Timing
- Review communication strategies relating to changes in policy/guidelines
- Review educational delivery
    - World Health Organization (WHO) check list
    - Blended learning an option

**Figure 8.11** Early Action Plan

## Conclusions

The best advice we can give at this point is to use the tool. The more you use it, the more information that you will gather as your experience increases. It sounds simple and obvious, but the more experienced practitioners the better the yield of information.

Having a mix of people conducting the investigation from various backgrounds adds to the value of the tool. They will have a focus that reflects their role. By having someone that is unfamiliar to the area or processes being looked at means that they will ask different questions and see different interactions.

Although the tool looks easy to use, it needs somebody to lead the conversation. This person can ensure that the interactions can be identified, otherwise all that is obtained is a list of factors. This would probably sit with the lead investigator, someone who has experience in Human Factors tools and methodology and has completed the PSIRF mandated investigative training. The gold standard would be to have a dedicated Human Factors practitioner in each Trust who could support the investigation team in application of systems-based tools such as AcciMap.

The AcciMap is a good tool to use to introduce systems thinking. It is great for staff to be able to look up and out at an incident as the different levels introduce different thoughts and factors. We are planning on providing our staff with some additional training on different aspects of the investigation process but do not feel that AcciMap needs further training.

There needs to be a discussion about the reporting chains for when external factors are identified. This probably needs a board-to-board level discussion and may reside with the Integrated Care Boards in the first instance.

Our next step is to make the transition from using it as a teaching tool to using it in 'real life' for the first time. We are looking for opportunities to use the new tools in the investigation of an incident.

## Reflections from the Frontline

- The tools identified highlight the complexity of healthcare work, and the challenges that have been faced in the past with trying to identify causes of harm without understanding the whole system.
- The fact that the case studies presented here were not examples of AcciMaps being used in a 'live' incident (one was research-based and one was training-based) demonstrates that AcciMaps are fairly new to investigations in healthcare. There have been discussions at the Patient Safety Management Network meetings about the use of AcciMaps but we don't have case study examples to share.

- The appearance of the completed AcciMaps could be off-putting to those who are asked to be involved in the investigation and forward actions process. The development of the AcciMap needs to be led by someone with a level of knowledge and skills in Human Factors. This may be a challenge for some organisations, although this gap is starting to close in healthcare with the introduction of the Patient Safety Syllabus, the role of the Patient Safety Specialists and PSIRF.
- What is also clear is that to use the tools successfully requires a significant amount of training and ongoing support to ensure that accurate learning is identified. There is a risk that if investigators try to use these tools without adequate training, then the findings identified may not be accurate. Appropriate training and development time should be given to anyone aiming to use these tools.

# References

Branford, K., Naikar, N. and Hopkins, A. (2009). 'Guidelines for Accimap analysis' in Hopkins, A. (ed.) *Learning from High Reliability Organisation.*, Sydney, Australia: CCH.

Carayon, P. *et al.* (2006). 'Work system design for patient safety: the SEIPS model' in *BMJ Quality & Safety*, 14; pp. i50–i58.

Goncalves Filho, A.P., Jun, G.T. and Waterson, P. (2019). 'Four Studies, Two Methods, One Accident — an Examination of the Reliability and Validity of Accimap and STAMP for Accident Analysis' in *Safety Science*, 113; pp. 310–317.

Healthcare Safety Investigation Branch (2020). *Placement of nasogastric tubes.* https://www.hssib.org.uk/patient-safety-investigations/placement-of-nasogastric-tubes/.

Hollnagel, E. (2004). *Barriers and Accident Prevention*. Aldershot: Ashgate Publishing.

Igene, O.O. *et al.* (2017). 'Is the Accimap Method an effective approach for analysing Adverse Events in the National Health Service, Scotland?' *48th Annual Conference of the Association of Canadian Ergonomists / 12th International Symposium on Human Factors in Organisational Design and Management*, pp. 448–455.

Igene, O.O. and Johnson, C. (2019). 'Analysis of medication dosing error related to Computerised Provider Order Entry system: A comparison of ECF, HFACS, STAMP and Accimap approaches' in *Health Informatics Journal*, 26(2); pp. 1017–1042. https://doi.org/10.1177/1460458219859992.

Igene, O.O. and Johnson, C. (2020). 'To Computerised Provider Order Entry system: A comparison of ECF, HFACS, STAMP and Accimap approaches' in *Health Informatics Journal*, 26(2); pp. 1017–1042.

Kee, D. (2017). 'Comparison of Systemic Accident Analysis Investigation Techniques Based on the Sewol Ferry Capsizing' in *Journal of the Ergonomics Society of Korea*, 36(5); pp. 485–498.

Leveson, N. (2004). 'A new accident model for engineering safer systems' in *Safety Science*, 42; pp. 237–270.

Murray, S., Waterson, P. and Jun, G.T. (2017). 'Collisions at sea: A systems analysis of causal factors and countermeasure' in Charles, R. and Wilkinson, J. (eds.) *Contemporary Ergonomics & Human Factors*. Chartered Institute of Ergonomics and Human Factors. https://publications.ergonomics.org.uk/uploads/Collisions-at-Sea-A-Systems-Analysis-of-Causal-Factors-and-Countermeasures.pdf.

NHS Education for Scotland (In Press). *Guidance on Accimaps for Safety Incident Investigations and Learning in Health and Social care.*

NHS England and NHS Improvement (2020). *Identifying patient safety specialists*. https://www.england.nhs.uk/publication/identifying-patient-safety-specialists/.

Rasmussen, J. (1997). 'Risk Management in a dynamic society: A modelling problem' in *Safety Science*, 27(2–3); pp. 183–213.

Rasmussen, J. and Svedung, I. (2000). *Proactive Risk Management in a Dynamic Society*. Swedish Rescue Services Agency. Karlstad, Sweden.

Salmon, P.M., Cornelissen, M. and Trotter, M.J. (2012). 'Systems-based accident analysis methods: A comparison of Accimap, HFACS, and STAMP' in *Safety Science*, 50; pp. 1158–1170. https://doi.org/10.1016/j.ssci.2011.11.009.

Svedung, I. and Rasmussen, J. (2002). 'Graphic representation of accident scenarios: mapping system structure and the causation of accidents' in *Safety Science,* 40; pp. 397–417. https://doi.org/10.1016/S0925-7535(00)00036-9.

Underwood, P. and Waterson, P. (2014). 'Systems thinking, the Swiss Cheese Model and accident analysis: A comparative systemic analysis of the Grayrigg train derailment using the ATSB, Accimap and STAMP models' in *Accident Analysis and Prevention,* 68; pp. 75–94. https://doi.org/10.1016/j.aap.2013.07.027.

Underwood, P., Waterson, P. and Braithwaite, G. (2016). '"Accident investigation in the wild" — A small-scale, field-based evaluation of the STAMP method for accident analysis' in *Safety Science,* 82; pp. 129–143.

Waterson, P.E. *et al.* (2017). '"Remixing Rasmussen": The evolution of Accimaps within systemic accident analysis' in *Applied Ergonomics,* 59(B); pp. 483–503.

Wheway, J. (2020). *Systems Models for Patient Safety: utility and usability for multiple incident analysis. MSc for Human Factors for Patient Safety.* Loughborough University. (Shared via personal communication.)

Wheway, J.L. and Jun, G.T. (2021). 'Adopting systems models for multiple incident analysis: utility and usability' in *International Journal for Quality in Health Care,* 33(4), mzab135.

Wiegmann, D.A. and Shappell, S.A. (2001). *A Human Error Analysis of Commercial Aviation Accidents Using the Human Factors Analysis and Classification System.* (HFACS). Virginia: U.S. Department of Transportation.

Wiegmann, D.A. and Shappell, S.A. (2003). *A Human Error Approach to Aviation Accident Analysis – The Human Factors Analysis and Classification System.* Aldershot: Ashgate Publishing.

Woodier, N. (2017). *Integrating ergonomics and human factors into healthcare incident investigation: using models from industry.* Independent Scholarship in Ergonomics, University of Derby. (Shared via personal communication.)

## Reading

British Standards Institution (2018). BS EN ISO 9241-11. *Ergonomics of human-system interaction. Part 11: Usability: definitions and concepts.* London: British Standards Institution.

Cambridge Dictionary (2021). definition of utility. Available at: Cambridge Dictionary, English Dictionary, Translations & Thesaurus. Cambridge: Cambridge University Press.

Goode, N. *et al.* (2016). 'Designing system reforms: Using a systems approach to translate incident analyses into prevention strategies' in *Frontiers in Psychology,* 7(DEC), pp. 1–17. https://doi.org/10.3389/fpsyg.2016.01974.

Isherwood, P. and Waterson, P. (2021). 'To err is system; a comparison of methodologies for the investigation of adverse outcomes in healthcare' in *Journal of Patient Safety and Risk Management,* 26(2); pp. 64–73. https://doi.org/10.1177%2F2516043521990261.

Salmon, P.M. *et al.* (2020). 'The big picture on accident causation: A review, synthesis and meta-analysis of Accimap studies' in *Safety Science,* 126. https://doi.org/10.1016/j.ssci.2020.104650.

Waterson, P.E. (2009). 'A critical review of the systems approach within patient safety research' in *Ergonomics,* 52(10); pp. 1185–1195.

Waterson, P.E. (2020). 'Causation, levels of analysis and explanation in systems ergonomics — a closer look at the UK NHS Morecambe Bay Investigation' in *Applied Ergonomics,* 84. https://doi.org/10.1016/j.apergo.2019.103011.

Waterson, P.E. *et al.* (2019). 'The Hospital Survey on Patient Safety Culture (HSPSC): a systematic review of the psychometric properties of sixty-two international studies' in *BMJ Open 9(e026896).* https://bmjopen.bmj.com/content/9/9/e026896.full.

Watt, A., Jun, G.T. and Waterson, P.E. (2019). 'Resilience in the blood transfusion process: everyday adaptations to "normal" work' in *Safety Science,* 120; pp. 498–505. https://doi.org/10.1016/j.ssci.2019.07.028.

CHAPTER 9

# Transformative Simulation
## To Patient Safety and Beyond

*Philip Gurnett, Sharon Weldon, Ken Spearpoint and Andy Buttery*

## Summary

This chapter explores uses of simulation beyond its more traditional educational applications, in areas such as design, redesign, investigation and more. It considers the research base and the advantages and disadvantages of using simulation in this context, including the challenges. It identifies how simulation has been used and benefits other industries, with a focus on safety, and finally how simulation can be used to create more effective and safe systems, processes and better service user experiences.

## Background

Healthcare simulation has an extensive history and relationship with patient safety. Healthcare simulation has been documented as far back as the Roman Empire (Owen, 2016). In the seventeenth century developments in medicine as a science drove an interest in anatomy and dissection that subsequently became an important component of teaching medicine. This led to the use of cadavers for dissection, and while many bodies were those of convicted criminals, there were not enough to meet training needs. This was exacerbated by a decrease in the number of death sentences at that time (Mitchell *et al.*, 2011). Sadly, this led to the rise of the body snatchers and a rather dark but evolutionary time for medicine and healthcare. As an alternative, the use of wax to provide anatomically correct models also evolved at this time (Schnalke, 1995). This became fundamental in teaching, alongside dissection, which is still used in modern medical education today.

During the twentieth century, with the development of modern technologies, models evolved into manikins that ranged from simple figures to those that were more complex with moving mechanical parts. The rapid increasing power and availability of computers led to further developments that have manifested in the multi-functional manikins we have today. All these developments had a focus on the practitioner learning either a skill or part of a skill. This is important to note in the context of patient safety as the move away from practising on patients was partly an ethical one (Issenberg and Scalese, 2008). Simulation provides an opportunity to practice procedures and processes in a secure environment prior to delivery to patients. While we question the ethics of 'practising' clinical procedures on patients, we have not yet questioned testing systems, processes, improvements and changes out on patients without first simulating them and understanding how this ultimately affects patients and other participants, including staff, and other systems, or how they could contribute to them.

In 2004, David Gaba described simulation as a technique not a technology. He described how simulation can be a driver for patient safety, and how it can be used from an educational perspective across numerous dimensions from competence to performance and team behaviours

(Gaba, 2004). Aggarwal *et al.* (2010) describe simulation as a training tool to improve patient safety, moving away from the assumption of experience equalling proficiency towards a model of demonstration of proficiency. Although neither Gaba nor Aggarwal explicitly suggest that simulation had a role outside of a learning modality, the Covid-19 pandemic highlighted its potential across the world with Health Education England (2020) embracing the role of simulation as part of a wider development suite for systems and work design.

This use is not new and has somewhat developed organically due to evolving needs. In 1989, Simon *et al.* (1989) described the use of a major incident simulation, the Beilinson hospital exercise, to evaluate how the hospital would cope in such a situation. It is important to note that the process was not intended to test delivery of patient care by individual teams. During the 1990s, the use of *in situ* simulation training by resuscitation teams evolved to also identify and address latent threats to enable safer teamworking (Capelle and Paul, 1996). During the early 2010s, Price *et al.* (2012) described the use of simulation to better understand the challenges of responding to major haemorrhage emergencies in the operating room. They identified environmental concerns, including too many people attending, non-technical skills, leadership and followership, by testing the system. They combined their approach with the need to develop the skills of participants in such emergency simulations.

Simulation techniques have also been used by others to test equipment, processes and teams. McLellan (1999) described the use of simulation to practice, test and develop trauma team processes. Power *et al.* (2019) demonstrated the use of simulation on a human patient simulator to test equipment designed to detect early deterioration in ventilated patients prior to its use clinically. This approach enabled them to identify any potential errors or flaws in the equipment they were looking to use.

Expansion beyond a pedagogical approach has driven the focus extensively outside the combined educational and developmental tool which Gaba (2004) described, in which the purpose was, essentially, training to address knowledge, skills, attitudes or behaviour. Use of simulation outside of education appears to have been somewhat slow; however, it has been undertaken outside of (and perhaps unnoticed by) the health and care education field but still within healthcare. Oh *et al.* (2008) described the use of simulation to investigate audio tone guidance in cardiopulmonary resuscitation (CPR), while Johnsen and Bolle (2008) also used simulation with a resuscitation theme: to understand how video communication with people calling for help can contribute to improving patient outcomes. Both examples have a focus on improvement of practice within their field with the use of simulation, outside of an '*in situ*' setting, to develop new processes. In both cases these techniques have evolved and become more broadly used.

The Covid-19 pandemic led to an international use of simulation within healthcare to design and test systems and processes. Simultaneously, but without any coordination or formal collaboration, simulation teams around the world stepped forward to assist with the systems design, redesign and personnel training, highlighting the valuable role simulation could provide outside of the educational frame. Brazil *et al.* (2020) used translational simulation methods (Brazil, 2017) as part of their preparations with hospital services in Australia. Meanwhile, Wong *et al.* (2021) detailed the development of a programme to train airway management during the pandemic in the UK. This ensured that the participants were better prepared to perform the essential skills despite the constraints related to the use of increased personal protective equipment (PPE) and meeting the requirements of upskilling a large number of practitioners quickly. While this was happening, Sharar-Chami *et al.* (2020), based in Lebanon, reported their use of the SHELL Human Factors model (Molloy *et al.*, 2005, Hawkins, 1994) to train healthcare practitioners and also to help identify latent threats to practice in the development of their protocols. This widespread use of simulation within healthcare, to not only educate but to understand and develop ways of working, has propelled the use of simulation beyond the boundaries of pedagogy.

## Simulation in Other Industries

Simulation is used in other industries to understand how systems interact, how they function, and how people working within the physical or theoretical interact with them and each other (Pedersen, 2012). Simulation can be used to understand the variety of human work (Shorrock, 2016) and the interplay between them together with better understanding of the seven archetypes of work that Shorrock (2017) went on to describe.

Pilots have been using simulators since the invention of flight. They are an invaluable tool for practising in an environment that ensures that they are safe both physically and psychologically. Although it is not possible to train for all eventualities, common factors can be addressed (Landman, 2018). Simulation familiarises pilots with the layout of their cockpits (Proctor and Van Zandt, 2008) informed by further understanding of the cognitive analysis, priorities, and interaction of humans with humans and systems. Simulation also allows them to practise their emergency procedures. However, to learn to fly, practical experience remains part of a pilot's training.

Like the airline industry, the nuclear industry uses simulation for training. Indeed, the organisation EDF Energy describe their nuclear reactor engineers as pilots (Fauquet-Alekhine, 2012) and provide simulation on full-scale simulators (Fauquet-Alekhine and Labrucherie, 2012) giving the operators of the complex safety-critical equipment opportunity to practise and understand how they work and how they contribute to the wider system.

These are just some examples of the use of simulation outside of healthcare, demonstrating elements of the alignment to our traditional perception within healthcare of simulation as a learning tool, and the use of simulation to design, redesign and investigate systems and processes. One commonality seen in other industries is the application of HFE experts in conjunction with the professionals working within the area. Their work, using a variety of methods, including simulation, is vital to understand how we interact on a person-to-person level and also with the complexity of our work.

## Human Factors and Ergonomics (HFE) and Its Link to Transformative Simulation

Simulation is one of the tools of the HFE practitioner. For example, Stanton *et al.* (2013) discussed the use of simulation as part of the assessment of mental workload, the Instantaneous Self-Assessment Method (ISA). Within this process, task analysis is undertaken normally with the use of simulation. In multiple HFE methods, task analysis is integral, and simulation is a way — often the optimum — to undertake this. It enables the practitioner to see what happens and question it. This questioning and use of simulation helps to understand the archetypes of work described by Shorrock (2017) and the 'messy reality' in particular. Across healthcare, opportunities for observation, particularly of a rarely performed or personally invasive procedure, is limited. Barriers include rarity and unpredictability, out-of-hours, reluctance from patients — and staff — to give consent and/or challenges to asking for consent. Simulation facilitates planned, timely, safe events ensuring better understanding with unconstrained opportunities to observe, test variations and generally freely explore without issues of consent or safety in a risk-managed process. However, the simulation will be an approximation (though meaningful) and not precisely the 'work done', as described by Hollnagel *et al.* (2006). This is where the debriefing element of healthcare simulation is vital to understand the participants' perceptions, emotions and, thus, their behaviours.

Transformative simulation is also vital in enabling the inclusion and involvement of the silent partners in healthcare that may be forgotten in our quest to improve a process or task. There are several issues that could be a barrier to further development of simulation outside of education. As already described, its role has been used for decades by healthcare practitioners who wanted to explore and understand their world. Most of this has been intuitive and a lot outside of professional fields, but to share this work has been either difficult or not thought worthy as it's 'just what we do'. The use outside of the educational modes does lead to the need for more guidance in how to do this. Of note is the work of Brazil (2017) in the development of the translational simulation methods. This approach, using simulation to identify, challenge and redesign systems and processes, provides one framework to use simulation.

We observe that a significant barrier to sharing and developing this work has been the constraints to meet publishers' requirements to record activity within accepted frameworks that force interventions to look like pedagogy. This significantly limits the opportunities for non-pedagogic simulation to be published, and, when it is, broadcast across the entire panoply of journals, unlikely to be easily found by those who would benefit. Therefore, a framework to guide the field is needed and this is what transformative simulation can add.

## The Transformative Simulation Taxonomy

Transformative simulation is used to describe the use of simulation to transform health and care through collective understanding, insight and learning as opposed to pedagogical approaches that are more commonly associated with simulation in healthcare (Weldon *et al.*, 2023). The term was developed as a result of an extensive literature review, and engagement with simulation communities of practice. The development of a taxonomy, a set of names and descriptions that are used to organise information in such a way that it is easier to access and share knowledge (Lambe, 2007), was generated to help to address the challenges of sharing practice and knowledge.

The objectives of any simulation are the starting point for designing scenarios and events and are fundamental to simulation design more generally (Hellaby, 2013; Issenberg *et al.*, 2005). This does not change when using simulation for systems testing, patient care design processes or investigative approaches. It is vital to have an overarching focus on what you wish to achieve. This is where the transformative simulation taxonomy helps to articulate a focus but also empowers curiosity for the unknown. While you have an overarching focus, you are still open to the potential unknowns that could be identified in the simulation or debriefing process.

The umbrella term 'transformative simulation' is made up of seven simulation-based 'Is' (SBI) described by Weldon *et al.* (2023) that give the designer a focus on what they want the simulation to achieve:

**Innovation:** The introduction of something new or a new way of doing things. This could be a technique for patient care, policy or a new system of work.
**Improvement:** Using simulation to contribute to the development of something that already exists, such as an established service.
**Intervention:** Contributes to changing a situation or way of doing things. For example, providing a risk-managed opportunity to disrupt an accepted process.
**Involvement:** Invites and engages others that may not normally participate or would otherwise have been excluded, with the purpose of generating new experience, building bridges and understanding between stakeholders. For example, providing a risk-managed opportunity for innovative public participation. The collaborative inclusion of patient/public participation is expected as part of involvement.
**Identification:** The use of simulation to understand what may be happening in a given situation, identifying latent threats and/or error producing design issues — both physical and systems based.

**Inclusion**: Relates to simulation that invites key stakeholders to share, empower and provide a platform for them to inform and reform relevant elements of health and social care.

**Influence**: Is the use of simulation to exert influence on someone or something. This can be through demonstration using simulation or may be through presentation of information from a simulation to those who can make change happen.

Although some of these are closely aligned to each other and may overlap, they each have a unique identity and can stand alone as a sole SBI.

These SBIs have been informed by the literature, meetings and workshops, with representatives of the simulation community through online and in-person events, held as part of wider simulation association conferences. This has been augmented through scholarly activity and literature reviews that demonstrate how the SBIs have been used for a significant period of time within healthcare, often in isolation and reported in outlier publications.

The SBIs are helpful in that they identify the overarching objectives of what the simulation is intended to explore. Taking objectives out of the educational and clinical context and language opens up the events that are being designed, empowers a freer framing of the role simulation has, and encourages empowered participation of all stakeholders. This is vital when simulation is being taken out of a clinical and/or educational context and into an area of health and care where the terminology and technology of clinical simulation is alien and could be a barrier to engagement.

In their application, SBIs provide a structural and functional starting point. It is important to be aware, and the taxonomy stresses this, that you may have more than one SBI focus. This is fine, as is the case in educational simulation where you may have multiple objectives. However, within transformative simulation they may be more easily distinguished as primary and secondary objectives for ease of design. For example, you may set out to *identify* the latent threats in a new clinical area but also plan to *influence* the use of simulation routinely for these purposes in a wider scope within an organisation so that it is used more effectively and becomes part of the design processes from the beginning. As a result of this, a second round of simulation might see you contributing to redesign as both an *improvement* and *intervention* but, using your knowledge of SBIs, you could also plan to *include* and *involve* stakeholders in this process.

Once you have identified the SBI(s) that will form your focus (and this may merit thoughtful attention), you can then work to design your simulation. This will involve collaborative approaches and may be a small part of a wider evolutionary or developmental process that, for example, includes information and co-design with ergonomists, information identified from sources such as SEIPS (see Chapter 3 on SEIPS) analysis and a quality improvement team (Carayon *et al.*, 2006). In the planning stages, SBIs may also benefit from being informed, in an integrated way, by more familiar project management processes, for example, Strengths, Weaknesses, Opportunities and Threats (SWOT) analysis (Heinz, 1982) and Plan, Do, Study, Act (PDSA) improvement cycles (Deming, 2000). Like educational simulation, the simulationist brings their expertise in the use of simulation to the process and will need collaboration with subject matter experts to help inform the design of the simulation. In addition to these traditional input approaches, the inclusion and involvement of SBIs can help to promote the collaboration of all stakeholders.

## Application

Figure 9.1 shows how applying simulation may look as a process. This is an example of an approach from the author's (PG) experience of using simulation to develop and change practice; however, there is more than one method to follow, notably the translational simulation approach (Brazil, 2017), and others identified in the literature in the transformative simulation taxonomy paper (Weldon *et al.*, 2023). Ultimately, there is no constraint against creating your own path. Undoubtedly, new SBI pathways will emerge as we learn from its application and find it easier to report and share experiences and subject this to peer review in a comparative literature environment.

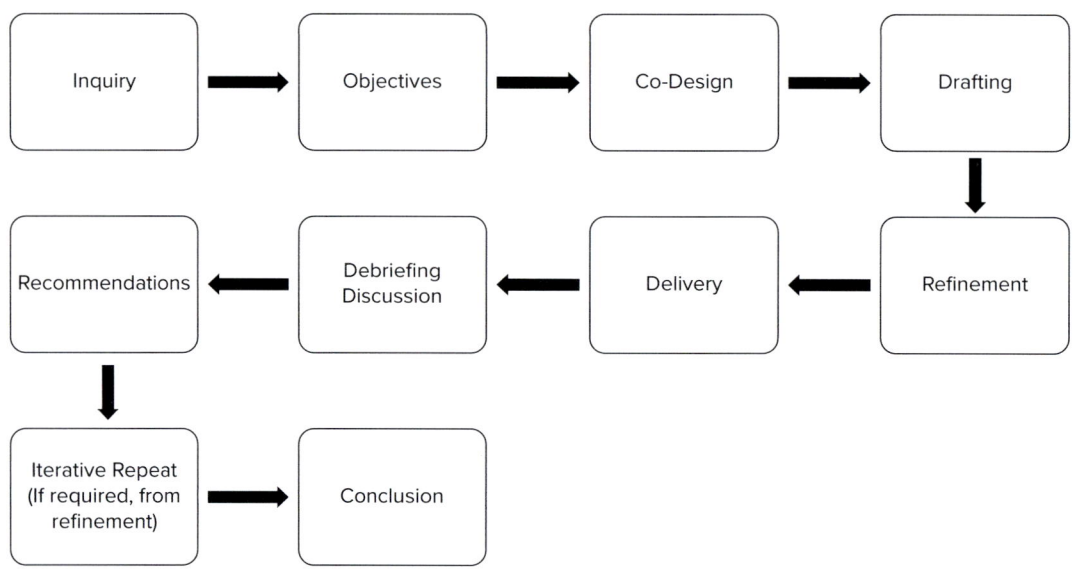

**Figure 9.1** Process for Applying Transformative Simulation

While the focus of this chapter has been largely on what transformative simulation can do and how, the true starting point would be the request for assistance. To the authors' knowledge there are no simulation services within UK practice that use a proactive structured SBI approach towards service improvement; they are more likely to be approached with a request to assist. With UK healthcare simulation funding largely supported from an educational perspective based on pedagogic outcomes, this evolving role may be challenging for simulation services. Transformative simulation can help us to move beyond the limitations of learning outcomes as measures.

The **inquiry** stage can be formal or informal. All of the authors have experienced the evolution of a simulation intervention from informal discussions as a starting point. The TS framework helps to provide a structured approach to begin the process. Most NHS hospitals will have simulation-based education teams that may be approached, however, these are currently not funded or resourced specifically to support this type of work and the need to collaboratively work with system and organisational support is paramount.

Identification of the **objectives** becomes the second stage. This is where the SBIs are identified to help inform and guide the further development. This process is likely to be iterative.

The third step of the process is the **co-design** stage. This incorporates the information gathering and will take into account the input from a variety of sources and could be dependent on the primary SBI that you are working with. For instance, you could be working on an Inclusion or Involvement and, therefore, it would be advantageous to include stakeholders in the co-design phase. You may be working as part of an Improvement and have input from a SEIPS analysis. Whatever your focus, the co-design stage uses the information gained to inform the drafting process. The importance in this phase is on the 'co' part of co-design. From a transformative approach, this is important as it will lead to a simulation that has more meaning for all participating with the knowledge that they/their group had been represented in the design and were not being stereotyped by the designers, or their role being seen as tokenistic or an add-on.

It is important to understand how the intended/imagined outcomes and the consequences/output that emerges during the running of the simulation is going to be captured, documented, and reported during the debrief, and by whom. Addressing these aspects in the planning phase will inform the focus of the team delivering the transformative simulation event and is critical to the quality of the event.

The **drafting** phase calls on all contributors to the design process to work together with the simulation team so that what is simulated is what had been imagined. This is similar to the development of clinical scenarios and consultation with subject matter experts in the clinical specialty being simulated.

The fifth phase, **refinement**, sees the simulation presented and piloted, and any refinement undertaken. This allows the co-contributors to have an understanding of what the simulation may look like. Piloting, while not only being good practice (INACSL, 2021) in a simulation also allows for changes and manipulations that may help you better understand what you are delivering.

**Delivery** of the simulation is the sixth phase. This will be specific to the scenario developed. The timeline for this will depend completely on what you want to achieve and how much detail or development is required for the simulation event. The inclusion of participants with little or no simulation experience will require more time to orientate to the process being used. Equally, simulation that is delivered collaboratively will need clear explanation to all participants. The fundamental principles of simulation delivery are still required, regardless of the reasoning behind the delivery.

The seventh phase within a transformative approach is a structured post-event **debriefing discussion**. This will loosely follow a debriefing structure and process. The techniques of a skilled simulation debriefer will be necessary to elicit perceptions of what has happened, opinions, experiences and evaluations in relation to the SBIs. There are two variations from a more traditional simulation-based education debriefing process.

Firstly, the participants may not have any knowledge of simulation, and they may not have any knowledge of healthcare, but their experience of the simulation or what it elicits for them is still valid and owned by them. This means that the facilitators need to be aware and willing to modify their approaches to elicit the experiences (simulation or recall-based). The facilitator must suppress the knowledge they have and be open to the opinions of those who have a differing view from a different perspective than the healthcare professional and/or the facilitator.

Secondly, while the closure approach of most inquiry-based debriefing models is about the participants' take home messages (Oriot and Alinier, 2018), within transformative simulation the take home messages are also for the team facilitating and observing the process being simulated. This may be the same as those who have participated but not always; it needs to be made clear at the beginning of the simulation that this is not an educational event but their contribution may lead to the education of others.

Once the structured discussion has been completed, the eighth stage is that of sharing the observations and **recommendations** with the wider investigators. This could be as part of a discussion or a formal report process. This dissemination of findings should be in a form that records the observations/recommendations with rationale and action points to be referred to and possibly used in the next stage. It is important that participants are aware that observations will be shared and to ensure that participants' confidentiality is maintained. The creation of the safe space is still a valid and expected requirement with transformative simulation. The fiction contract (Dieckmann, 2009; Rudolph *et al.*, 2014) must be worked at by the facilitators of the simulation, often with more depth.

Simulation design is an **iterative** process with the need to continually adapt and update. There may be a requirement for a ninth stage to be undertaken. Refinement from the information already gained informs a repeat of the simulation to ensure any recommendations work as imagined. Once this has been completed, move to the final stage.

Finally, at the tenth stage, **conclusions**, the summarised observations are shared with the wider stakeholders involved in the process. It is also a chance to reflect and identify how you would develop your processes further.

This approach can appear time consuming but has several advantages. The ten steps break down the overall process into easily manageable segments that allow facilitators to better understand where they are within the process. This demonstrates progress and allows focus on what needs to happen to complete the process.

Following this process also contributes to the succesful change characteristics that Nilsen *et al.* (2020) described where participants have a sense of being able to influence change, being part of the design process both within the simulation and the wider HFE approach.

# Conclusions

This chapter has taken the reader through the application of simulation for a non-pedagogical approach. We have explained the background to this and that, in reality, this is not a new use of simulation but is something that has been undertaken with little recognition of its worth within healthcare.

To deliver transformative simulations, there is a need for skilled simulationists and simulation teams to work collaboratively with stakeholders. This collaborative approach, together with support from organisations, can see transformative simulation not only contributing to safer working practices but also to truly holistically designed healthcare.

**CASE STUDY 1**

Emma Broughton, Head of Education for Simulation at a Tertiary Paediatric Hospital

## Background

In 2020, our organisation introduced a surgical procedure that was not previously offered by the Trust. Prior to the introduction of this care pathway, the simulation team were approached to conduct a 'run through' simulation exercise to assist the MDT involved in this procedure through rehearsal of the patient pathway between the hospital's neonatal unit and operating theatre.

The inquiry focused on transfer between the two care environments. This was deemed to be a high-risk aspect of the patient journey in recognition of the multiple teams involved, and the complexity of tasks associated with transfer to and from the theatre environment.

The simulation team advocated for a full-scale live simulation to accurately reflect the care pathway that this patient cohort would follow. Due to the number of teams involved in this procedure, and the nuances around internal transfers between acute environments, a large-scale exercise was deemed to be more appropriate than several siloed efforts focusing on segments of the patient's surgical care.

The exercise set out to use simulation to inform and influence the patient pathway and SOP for this procedure.

The following objectives were agreed as part of a joint needs assessment with the clinical teams:

### Innovation

- Rehearse the safe transfer of neonate from Neonatal Intensive Care Unit to Cardiac Cath Lab.
- Rehearse the set-up and walkthrough of a patent ductus arteriosus (PDA) closure procedure, including positioning of patient and all intra-operative equipment.

## Identification
- Troubleshoot the process for patient warming during transfer and surgical procedure.
- Navigate the proposed SOP for closure of neonatal PDA in the Cath Lab.

## What We Did

One month prior to the exercise, the simulation team met with key stakeholders to understand their aims for the exercise and to learn more about the proposed pathway for these patients as part of the co-design phase. Input from the clinical, surgical and anaesthetic teams formed the basis for the overarching objectives and focus of the exercise. A date was agreed for the following month based around theatre downtime. Each team took responsibility for securing the personnel, resources and space required to conduct the simulation, the drafting and refinement, accurately at each point of the patient pathway. Figures 9.2 and 9.3 show the simulation set-up.

The stakeholders included theatre team leaders, specialty leads, medical consultants and ward managers. These senior team members played a fundamental role in protecting time for staff to participate in the event. Early engagement was attributed to the fact that a regular *in situ* simulation provision was already embedded across the Trust, with buy-in from quality and safety leads as well as senior managers. Moreover, the simulation team formed part of a weekly safety committee, where latent errors identified through simulation were reported at a high level. Consequently, the use of simulation as a patient safety intervention was not a new concept for the teams involved and they were already open to a culture which embraced simulation.

Before this exercise, all latent errors captured via simulation were reported within a designated domain of the Trust incident reporting system. This meant that each latent error was reported and followed up separately in a bid to close the loop on each individual risk. As this was the first exercise of its kind, it was felt that a robust and detailed report would be required to prevent the outcomes from being siloed. Moreover, it was thought that a comprehensive report would ensure actions and recommendations were clearly defined and assigned to local action owners where appropriate.

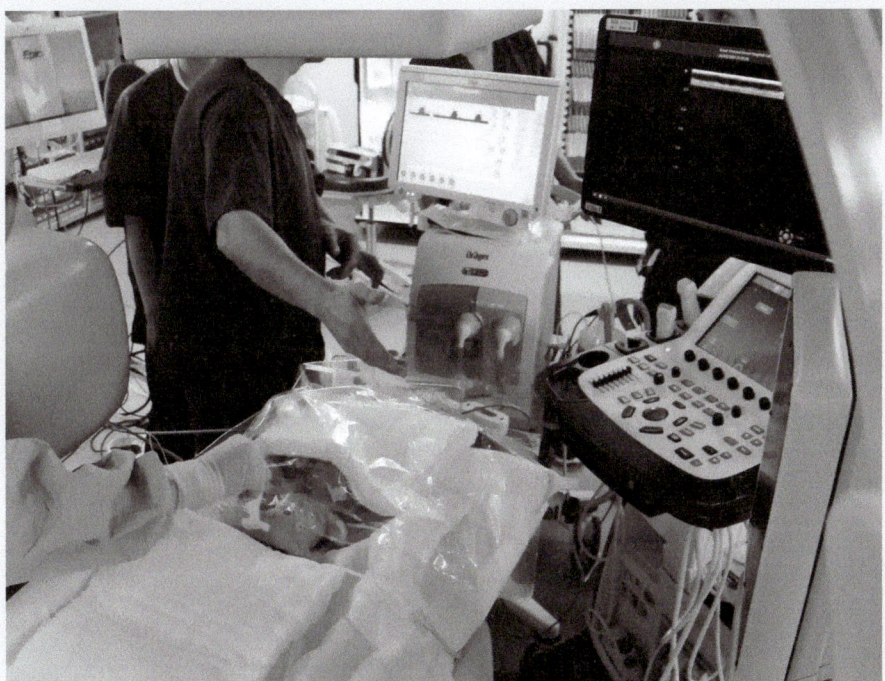

**Figure 9.2** Simulated Patient Being Prepped for Surgery

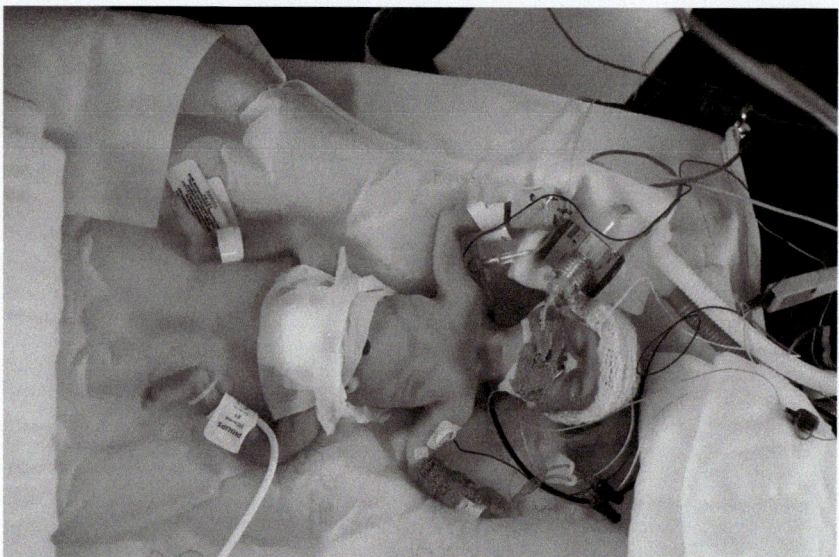

**Figure 9.3** Simulated Neonatal Set-up on the Operating Table

In seeking out an evidence-based structure for the findings of the simulation, the SEIPS model (Carayon *et al.*, 2006) was identified. During delivery and debrief, the observations from the exercise were mapped to the domains of SEIPS, which provided a useful structure for the session report. Recommendations or actions were assigned to each of the observations, based on the expert input offered by the team members involved.

## Lessons Learned

### What Worked Well?

We attributed the success of the exercise to several factors:

- Engagement and input from the clinical teams involved in this patient pathway.
- The opportunity to agree shared goals for the exercise.
- Effective communication with all parties involved.
- Buy-in and presence from senior team members.
- Local ownership of actions and recommendations.
- An open culture which enabled stakeholders to contribute.

The support of the medical consultants, theatre team leaders and clinical leads was central to the success of this exercise. Their engagement with the planning and delivery of this intervention role-modelled investment in simulation and a commitment to improving outcomes for patients. Furthermore, the exercise was framed as an opportunity to influence and improve the workflow. Anecdotally, this appeared to diffuse some of the anxiety that has previously been observed in response to simulation in these areas of practice. This highlighted the importance of clearly stating the aims and scope for the exercise during the pre-simulation brief.

### What Didn't Go So Well?

The timescale for the exercise proved to be the greatest challenge. Two hours of protected time had been allocated for the simulation; however, this extended to four hours. This created a potential risk to stakeholders by placing them under time pressure when they had clinical duties to attend to in preparation for the next day.

Although actions were captured as the event played out, the team were left with a 30-minute opportunity to debrief at the end of the exercise. The debrief was structured by returning to the initial objectives of the exercise while seeking reflections and feedback on each of these points.

Although this helped to draw out the outcomes from the simulation, with 18 participants present not everyone had the opportunity to comment due to the time constraints.

For these cases, parents or carers would usually be present during key moments of ward-based care. Despite this, representation from parents or carers was not considered. This may have been a missed opportunity to seek input from families to help shape aspects of the care pathway, such as checking out of the ward environment.

## Evaluation and Impact

From the exercise there was a total of 18 outcomes that led to recommendations for future practice. Many of these recommendations related to the physical environment, which was already established prior to the introduction of this new patient intervention. Other outcomes included modifiable factors around communication processes and availability of clinical equipment. A summary of the findings is shown in Figure 9.4 mapped to the domains of SEIPS.

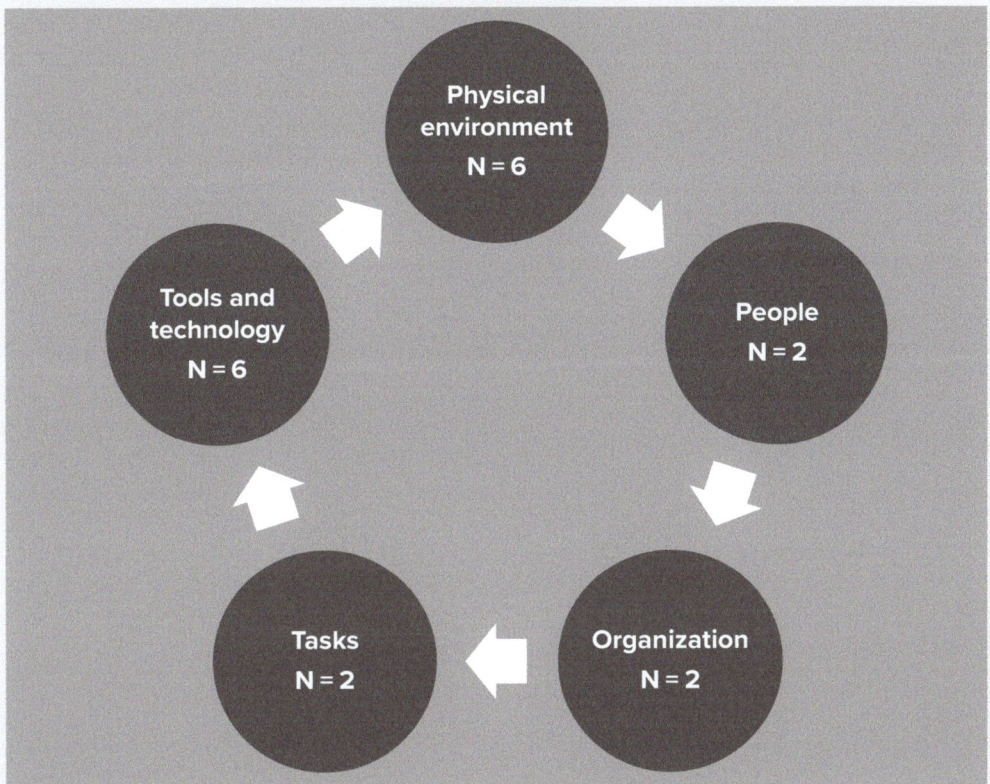

Figure 9.4 Outcomes Mapped to the Domains of SEIPS (2006)

Observations were noted throughout the duration of the exercise, with two facilitators capturing notes. The stakeholders were then taken back through the objectives and timeline of the patient pathway during the debrief and invited to feedback any additional observations or recommendations. These actions were then compiled into a report by the simulation team and shared with all participants.

Due to the nature and scope of this simulation, a standardised session evaluation was not deemed appropriate. Instead, team members were invited to comment on or add to the session report — as they were regarded as the subject matter experts in this case. On reflection, it would have been useful to understand their experience as experts and stakeholders, separate to the outcomes of the session. This is something that has since been implemented in subsequent similar exercises.

This exercise became the first of many applications of simulation to support systems integration within the organisation. Following the success of this initial endeavour, a further 20 exercises have been delivered with 79 latent errors captured and several protocols influenced. A snapshot of the subsequent exercises is provided in Figure 9.5.

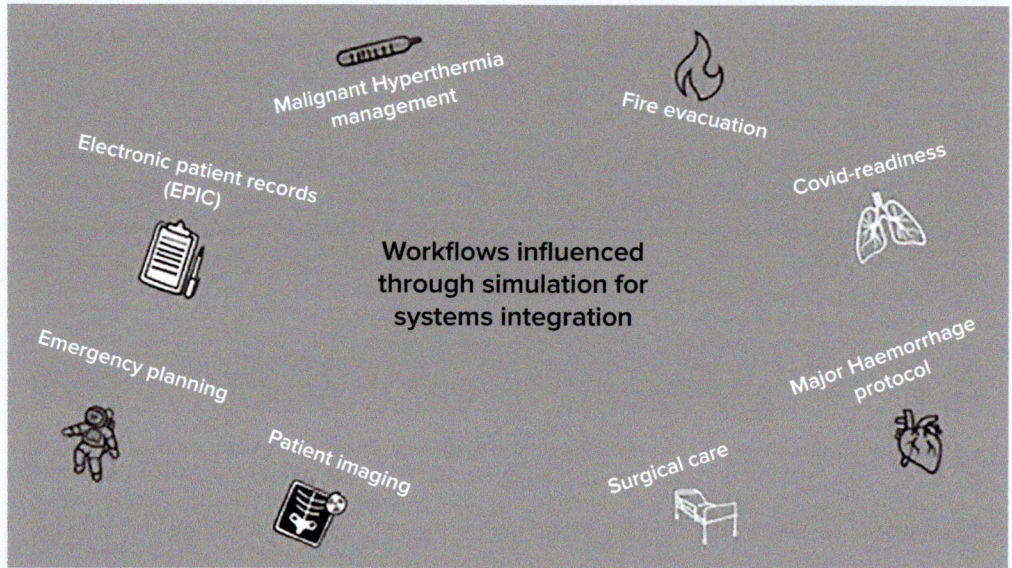

Figure 9.5 Workflows Influenced by Subsequent Simulations

Having input from families could have strengthened the outcomes of this simulation, given the unique insight they can provide from their lived experience. Further, there was only a short turn-around between the exercise taking place and the first patient being treated on this pathway. Had there been more time between these interventions, the simulation could have been revisited to assess the impact of the outcomes from the initial exercise.

## Conclusions

Key elements needed to establish a successful systems level simulation:

- Identify protected time for planning, delivery and follow-up.
- Ensure engagement from key stakeholders from the outset.
- Engage stakeholders in needs assessment.
- Invite stakeholders to set the aims and objectives.
- Seek high-level buy-in from the organisation.
- Identify a mechanism for reporting outcomes.
- Ensure local ownership of actions.
- Consider feasibility of repeating the simulation to enable evaluation of long-term impact.

The SEIPS model is traditionally used as a tool to examine system safety in the context of live workflows. In this case study, you could argue that the model was used beyond its intended scope by being applied retrospectively to analyse and structure findings. Although this approach proved to be an effective way of gleaning focused recommendations from the simulation, had the tool been used prospectively during the simulation, the team may have viewed the simulated workflow through a more focused lens.

The key learnings from the exercise were the value of early engagement from stakeholders; the need to protect adequate time for design, delivery, evaluation and dissemination; and the importance of a mechanism for reporting outcomes. Importantly, the output from this exercise helped to demonstrate the value of simulation to support systems integration. Consequently, this application of simulation has since seen significant growth across the organisation.

Since this simulation intervention was carried out, 15 patients have successfully been treated on this surgical pathway. Beyond the scope of the initial exercise, the following areas are currently being explored for future development:

- Use of the Promoting Excellence and Reflective Learning in Simulation (PEARLS) debrief model for systems integration exercises (Dubé *et al.*, 2019)
- Adopting an iterative approach to assess immediate and long-term impact of simulation interventions.
- Patient and family involvement in the design and delivery of simulation.
- Using simulation to support hospital transformation projects.

For the future, it is our aim to continue to raise the profile of simulation as a tool to enhance, influence and inform our hospital systems, making them safer for patients and workforce alike.

## Reflections from the Frontline

- The challenges in using this approach, as ever in simulation, include resources and, more specifically, capability to apply this type of simulation approach effectively. You need to engage, motivate and support participants to be part of something that doesn't follow the traditional expectations and outcome measures of simulation-based education.
- The simulation in the case study took four hours rather than two. This highlights the need for protected time to be allocated to not only carry out a simulation but allowing enough time for a debrief too. This can be difficult to get with frontline staff already under pressure.
- There needs to be 'buy-in' across the spectrum of organisations and participants involved prior to and during the simulation process being applied, similar to any processes and projects that necessitate change, and a willingness to act on the outcomes.
- The use of simulation, while not new within healthcare, requires facilitators, often from a healthcare profession background, who are willing to put aside their own informed personal views and apply their expertise in simulation, including analytic observation.
- Transformative simulation offers the opportunity to use simulation differently, with a different focus that encompasses not just patient safety but also the engagement with participants in health and care, engagement with persons that influence health and care, and engagement with systems and processes that impact health and care.
- In the case study, the parents were not involved, and this was a missed opportunity to seek input from them to help shape aspects of the care pathway and gain a different perspective and input.
- A move to develop faculty from outside of healthcare as facilitators could enhance the opportunities for transformative simulation and patient safety as a whole. Including the lay faculty (non-clinical people who are running the simulation) brings a voice to challenge what can often be an approach laden with assumptions within healthcare and simulation.

## References

Aggarwal R. *et al.* (2010). 'Training and simulation for patient safety' in *Quality and Safety in Health Care*, 19(Suppl 2): pp. 34–43.

Brazil, V. (2017). 'Translational Simulation: Not "where?" but "why?" A functional view of in situ simulation' in *Advances in simulation*, 2(20). https://doi.org/10.1186/s41077-017-0052-3.

Brazil, V. et al. (2020). 'Translational simulation for rapid transformation of health services, using the example of the COVID-19 pandemic preparation' in *Advances in Simulation,* 5(9). doi: 10.1186/s41077-020-00127-z.

Capelle, C. and Paul, R. (1996). 'Educating Residents: The effects of a mock code program' in *Resuscitation,* 31 pp. 107–111. doi: 10.1016/0300-9572(95)00919-1.

Carayon, P. et al. (2006). 'Work system design for patient safety: the SEIPS model' in *Quality and Safety in Health care,* Suppl 1, pp. i50–i58. doi: 10.1136/qshc.2005.015842.

Deming, W.E. (2000). *Out of the crisis.* Cambridge, MA: MIT Press.

Dieckmann, P. (2009). 'Simulation settings for learning in acute medical care' in *Using Simulation for education, training and research,* pp. 40–138. Lengerich: Pabst.

Dubé, M.M. et al. (2019). 'PEARLS for Systems Integration' in *Simulation in Healthcare: The Journal of the Society for Simulation in Healthcare,* 14(5): pp. 333–342. doi: 10.1097/sih.0000000000000381.

Fauquet-Alekhine, P. (2012). 'Simulation for training pilots of French nuclear power plants' in *Socio-Organizational Factors for Safe Nuclear Operation.* pp. 69–74. Montagret: Larsen Science Ed.

Fauquet-Alekhine, P. and Labrucherie, M. (2012). 'Simulation training debriefing as a work activity analysis tool. The case of nuclear reactor pilots and civil aircraft pilots' in *Socio-Organizational Factors for Safe Nuclear operations.* First edition, pp. 79–83. Montagret: Larsen Science.

Gaba, D. (2004). 'The future vision of simulation in healthcare' in *BMJ Quality and Safety,* 13(suppl 1) pp. i2–i10. doi: 10.1136/qhc.13.suppl_1.i2.

Hawkins, F.W. (1994). *Human Factors in flight.* Aldershot: Ashgate Publishing.

Health Education England (2020). *Enhancing education, clinical practice and staff wellbeing. A national vision for the role of simulation and immersive learning technologies in health and care.* Available at: https://www.hee.nhs.uk/sites/default/files/documents/National%20Strategic%20Vision%20of%20Sim%20in%20Health%20and%20Care.pdf

Heinz, W. (1982). 'The TOWS matrix — a tool for situational analysis' in *Long Range Planning,* 15(2): pp. 54–66. doi: 10.1016/0024-6301(82)90120-0.

Hellaby, M. (2013). *Healthcare Simulation in Practice.* Keswick: M&K Publishing.

Hollnagel, E., Woods, D.D. and Levison, N. (2006). *Resilience Engineering: Concepts and Precepts.* Aldershot: Ashgate Publishing.

INACSL Standards Committee, McDermott, D.S., Ludlow, J., Horsley, E. and Meakim, C. (2021). 'Healthcare Simulation Standards of Best Practice Pre-briefing: Preparation and Briefing' in *Clinical Simulation in Nursing,* 58, pp. 9–13. doi: 10.1016/j.ecns.2021.08.008.

Issenberg, B.S. et al. (2005). 'Features and uses of high-fidelity medical simulations that lead to effective learning: a BEME systematic review' in *Medical Teacher,* 27(1): pp. 10–28.

Issenberg, S.B. and Scalese, R.J. (2008). 'Simulation in health care education' in *Perspectives in Biology and Medicine,* 51(1): pp. 31–46.

Johnsen, E. and Bolle, S.R. (2008). 'To see or not to see — Better dispatcher-assisted CPR with video-calls? A qualitative study based on simulated trials' in *Resuscitation,* 78, pp. 320–326. doi: 10.1016/j.resuscitation.2008.04.024.

Lambe, P. (2007). *Organising knowledge: Taxonomies, knowledge and organisational effectiveness.* Woodhead: Chandos Publishing.

Landman A. et al. (2018). 'Pilots for unexpected events: A simulator study of the advantages of unpredictable and variable scenarios' in *Human Factors,* 60(6): pp. 793–805. doi: 10.1177/0018720818779928.

McLellan, B. (1999). 'Early Experience with Simulated Trauma Resuscitation' in *Cardiac Journal of Surgery,* 42(3): pp. 205–210. PMID: 10372017; PMCID: PMC3788951.

Mitchell, P.D. et al. (2011). 'The Study of Anatomy in England from 1700 to the early 20th Century' in *Journal of Anatomy,* 219, pp. 91–99. doi: 10.1111/j.1469-7580.2011.01381.x.

Molloy, Gerard J., O'Boyle and Ciarán A. (2005). 'The SHEL Model: A Useful Tool for Analyzing and Teaching the Contribution of Human Factors to Medical Error' in *Academic Medicine,* 80(2): pp. 152–155.

Nilsen, P. et al. (2020). 'Characteristics of successful changes in health care organizations: an interview study with physicians, registered nurses and assistant nurses' in *BMC Health Service Research,* 20: p. 147. doi: 10.1186/s12913-020-4999-8.

Oh, J.H. *et al.* (2008). 'Effects of audio tone guidance on performance of CPR in simulated cardiac arrest with an advanced airway' in *Resuscitation,* 79 pp. 273–277. doi: 10.1016/j.resuscitation.2008.06.022.

Oriot, D. and Alinier, G. (2018). *Pocket book of simulation debriefing in healthcare.* Cham: Springer.

Owen, H. (2016). *Simulation in Healthcare Education. An extensive history.* London: Springer.

Pedersen, S.B. (2012). 'Interactivity in health care: bodies, values and dynamics' in *Language Sciences,* 34. pp. 532–542.

Power, D. *et al.* (2019). 'Simulation Test: Can medical devices pass?' in *BMJ Simulation and Technology Enhanced Learning* 6(5): pp. 302–303. doi: 10.1136/bmjstel-2019-000519.

Price, J. *et al.* (2012). 'Code Blue emergencies. A team task analysis and educational initiative' in *Canadian Medical Journal,* 3(1): e4–e20. PMID: 26451171; PMCID: PMC4563641.

Proctor, R.W. and Van Zandt, T. (2018). *Human Factors in Simple and Complex Systems.* Oxfordshire, UK: Routledge.

Rudolph, J., Raemer, D. and Simon, R. (2014). 'Establishing a safety container for learning in simulation. The role of pre-simulation briefing' in *Simulation in Healthcare,* 9(6): pp. 336–349.

Schnalke, T. (1995). *Diseases in Wax. The history of the medical moulage.* Berlin: Quintessence Books.

Sharar-Chami, R. *et al.* (2020). 'In Situ Simulation. An essential tool for safe preparedness for the COVID-19 Pandemic' in *Simulation in Healthcare,* 15(5): pp. 303–309. doi: 10.1097/SIH.0000000000000504.

Shorrock, S. (2016). *The Varieties of Human Work. Humanistic Systems.* Available at: https://humanisticsystems.com/2016/12/05/the-varieties-of-human-work/.

Shorrock, S. (2017). *The Archetypes of Human Work:1 The Messy Reality. Humanistic Systems.* Available at: https://humanisticsystems.com/2017/01/13/the-archetypes-of-human-work/.

Simon, D. *et al.* (1989). 'A new method for simulated mass casualty evaluation: The Beilinson hospital exercise' in *Pre-hospital and Disaster Medicine,* 4(2): pp. 122–126. doi: 10.1017/S1049023X00029885.

Stanton, N.A. *et al.* (2013). *Human Factors Methods. A practical guide for engineering and design.* London: CRC Press.

Weldon, S. *et al.* (2023). 'Transformative Forms of Simulation in Healthcare — the seven simulation-based "I"s: A concept taxonomy review of the literature' in *International Journal of Healthcare Simulation,* pp. 1–13. doi: 10.54531/tzfd6375.

Wong, H.Y., Johnstone, C. and Dua, G. (2021). 'Developing a simulation programme to train airway management during the COVID-19 pandemic in a tertiary-level hospital' in *BMJ Simulation and technology enhanced learning,* 7(6): pp. 631–634. doi: 10.1136/bmjstel-2020-000755.

## Reading

Papadopoulou, T. (2020). 'Developing construction graduates fit for the 4th industrial revolution through fieldwork application of active learning' in *Higher Education Pedagogies,* 5(1): pp. 182–199. doi: 10.1080/23752696.2020.1816844.

Phelps, J.M. *et al.* (2018). 'Experiential Learning and Simulation-Based Training in Norwegian Police Education: Examining Body-Worn Video as a Tool to Encourage Reflection' in *Policing: A Journal of Policy and Practice,* 12(1): pp. 50–65. doi: 10.1093/police/paw014.

Raduntz, T. *et al.* (2020). 'Indexing mental workload during simulated air traffic control tasks my means of dual frequency head maps' in *Frontiers in Psychology,* 11(300). doi: 10.3389/fphys.2020.00300.

Rosetti, M.D., Trzcinski, G.F. and Syverud, S.A. (1999). 'Emergency Department Simulation and Determination of Optimal Attending Physician Staffing Schedules' in Farrington, F.A. *et al.* (eds.) *Proceedings of the 1999 Winter Simulation Conference,* pp. 1532–1540. doi: 10.1145/324898.325315.

Saus, E. *et al.* (2006). 'The Effect of Brief Situational Awareness Training in a Police Shooting Simulator: An Experimental Study' in *Military Psychology,* 18 (Suppl) S3-S21. doi: 10.1207/s15327876mp1803s_2.

Smith, R. (2010). 'The Long History of Gaming in Military Training' in *Simulation & Gaming,* 41(1): pp. 6–19. doi: 10.1177/1046878109334330.

Williams-Bell, F.M. *et al.* (2015). 'Using Serious Games and Virtual Simulation for Training in the Fire Service: A Review' in *Fire Technology,* 51, pp. 553–584. doi: 10.1007/s10694-014-0398-1.

CHAPTER **10**

# Thematic Reviews in Patient Safety

*Samantha Machen*

## Summary

Learning from when things go wrong in healthcare is a common and established aim of health systems around the world (Doupi, 2009). Whilst implicitly it seems like learning from things going wrong is rather simple, in reality it is much more complex than simply sharing individual cases or experience. Defining 'learning' in the context of patient safety is important — what do we want to get out of imparting the information? Do we think simply sharing information will affect future care? The barriers to learning from errors are well discussed in current literature, where researchers identify the multi-faceted and cultural barriers that may exist, and argue that ensuring learning from errors occurs is easier said than done (Shojania, 2009; Thomas & Petersen, 2003; Olsen, 2007). Safety science identifies that incidents should be used as a trigger to further investigation of the whole system, process or task. However, it has become commonplace for individual incidents to be the focus of investigations under certain patient safety agendas — for example, NHS organisations following the mandated Serious Incident (SI) framework.

This chapter presents the argument for thematic reviews of patient safety incidents, when they can be used, what they offer over individual incident investigations, the methodology that can be used and a worked example of a fictious themed review.

## Background

In the context of wider research, even beyond healthcare, thematic reviews or thematic analysis refers to an analytical method or tool used in qualitative research to analyse narrative data. Thematic analysis is referred to as 'a method for identifying, analysing, and interpreting patterns of meaning ('themes')' (Braun and Clarke, 2006) and has been a popular research method since the early twentieth century. Braun and Clarke's thematic analysis method provides a step-by-step iterative approach to analysis, which consists of six steps: (i) becoming familiar with the data; (ii) generating codes; (iii) generating themes; (iv) reviewing themes; (v) defining and naming themes; and (vi) locating exemplars (Braun and Clarke, 2006). By using these steps, large amounts of narrative data can be analysed, and cross-cutting themes are identified and reported on. Within healthcare, thematic analysis is routinely used for qualitative research — for example, within ethnographic studies or research into staff or patient experiences.

Thematic reviews within the context of patient safety as a concept is an applied use of this established and well-respected analytical method. Thematic reviews for patient safety incidents, and the focus of this chapter, refer to clustering patient safety incidents together and analysing them together to identify system failures and areas for improvement. While anecdotally this has been standard practice for some organisations across healthcare in the past, there has not been a set standard or method available to follow. For example, an organisation may look at a cluster of incidents across a year that pertain to the same issue — such as falls or pressure ulcers — and they may use narrative from the incident description to analyse all the incidents in the sample size. This data may also be analysed based on set criteria recorded; for example, time or location of incident. Crucially, all approaches to thematic reviews in patient safety are trying to identify common themes or 'trends' to aid learning.

Within the context of patient safety in the NHS, thematic reviews have been used but not encouraged by the investigatory standards set out in national frameworks. Since 2015, the SI framework encouraged a single-incident analysis technique and, up until 2022, this was the mandated investigatory approach for NHS-funded organisations. In August 2022, PSIRF was released by NHS England which replaces the SI framework. The PSIRF advocates for systems thinking and is based on safety science standards, and in the context of thematic reviews, it encourages multi-incident reviews. This has been an important move away from single-incident focus towards focus on multiple incidents to aid systems thinking and subsequent improvement. Safety science literature argues that a single incident focus is potentially ineffective due to an over-focus on a very small proportion of incidents (Macrae, 2015; Stavropoulou, *et al.*, 2015) and an assumption that systems and processes fail in the exact same way. The argument for thematic reviews will now be presented to pinpoint the opportunities that the reviews offer individuals working in patient safety, to aid identification of failures in systems and supplement subsequent improvement plans.

## The Argument for Thematic Reviews

Herbert Heinrich proposed an influential cornerstone of safety philosophy in the form of the accident triangle in the 1930s. Heinrich puts forward this model, seen in Figure 10.1, to identify the relationship between accidents and more latent unsafe acts or activities. The original vernacular used by Heinrich was accidents, but professionals in patient safety may now be more confident with the term incident over accident. The model, latterly added to by Frank Bird, was used to identify that for one fatality or high harm event, there would be multiple events that cause less harm or have lesser impact and many more occasions of no harm. Although the files used to confirm Heinrich's numbers have since been lost, there has been evidence to confirm that when using large data sets the ratios suggested by Heinrich, and latterly Bird, do hold up across safety critical industries (Health and Safety Executive, 1999).

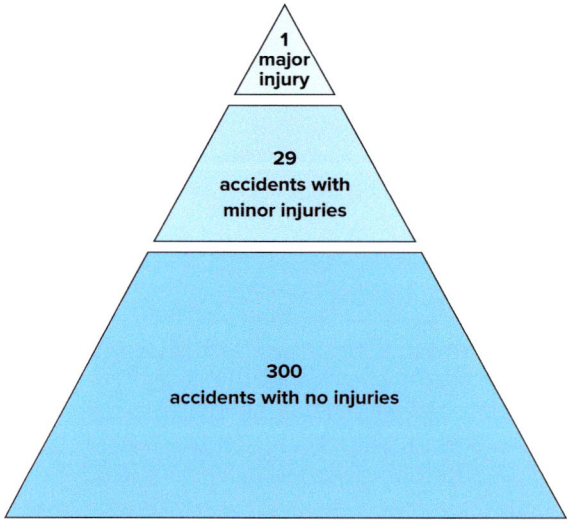

**Figure 10.1** Heinrich Model of the Accident Triangle

Moving the specific numbers aside, the model proposes a very important idea — that systems can fail multiple times but create different consequences. One system or task failure could result in a death, and another could be a narrow near miss. This is an important concept and one that is central to thematic reviews in patient safety. An applied example of this concept in patient safety may be in the context of the system of safety for management of a deteriorating patient.

Let us propose the system of safety, in a simple form, for managing a deteriorating patient:

1. Identification of patient at risk of deterioration.
2. Monitoring the patient's clinical condition (e.g. task of observation and monitoring National Early Warning Score (NEWS2)).
3. Escalation of any clinical deterioration (e.g. a high NEWS2 prompting nurse to refer patient to doctor for escalation).
4. Management of patient's deterioration (e.g. fluid resuscitation, antibiotics, any interventions needed).

Using the premise behind the accident triangle, we may identify one case of death or severe harm to a patient due to mismanagement of a patient's clinical condition. In this fictitious example, the patient has had a rising NEWS2 of 5 in the morning, increasing to 9 before getting septic shock and requiring interventional treatment in intensive care. Investigating this as an individual incident may highlight that, in this instance, there was a failure in the monitoring of this patient and there was a delay in doing observations for six hours, resulting in an action plan directly related to those issues. However, if we use the premise behind the accident triangle, we may delve into this system of safety slightly more deeply and look at the other incidents that may not result in high harms. We might be looking to cases where all four stages of the system of safety have failed, with differing outcomes. There may be cases where patients have had delays in initial assessment and, therefore, delaying identification of risk of deterioration (e.g. a patient presenting with sepsis in the emergency department (ED)). There may also be multiple cases of delays to observations resulting in no harm. There may also be examples of delays to escalation — for example, the absence of an automatic system that alerts outreach teams to high NEWS2 cases. Some of these cases may not have caused harm, some of them may have caused moderate harm, but what all these cases show us is that there are multiple issues across the whole four stages to this system of safety. (Degree of harm is defined by NHS England's Severity Mapping at www.england.nhs.uk/wp-content/uploads/2019/10/NRLS_Degree_of_harm_FAQs_-_final_v1.1.pdf.) Analysing the whole system of safety may allow us to create action plans and recommendations that focus on all parts of the system of work and any fallibilities identified. The argument for thematic reviews of incidents in patient safety rests upon the argument that a single incident focus may miss other cases where harm has not occurred, but the system has still failed and in another circumstance could have resulted in harm.

Systems of safety in healthcare are complex and, therefore, gaining as much insight into the way tasks and processes are operationalised and their impact on safety and quality is essential. Imagine if you were tasked with investigating the process of you getting to work on time based on one very unfortunate Monday morning where multiple things that usually run smoothly did not that day. Yes, you could focus solely on the case at hand, or you could look at the wider picture of what normally happens and how common these problems or disruptions are. If your car broke down on this unfortunate Monday morning, you might want to take a wider look at all the mornings you have been travelling to work in the past month and enquire as to whether there have been problems with your car regularly. If you look across 20 workday mornings and notice lots of near misses or signs that there were issues that still existed but that did not ultimately affect your time to set off, then this may help you build a bigger picture as to the scale of the problem. Similarly, if you looked at 20 workday mornings and noted this was the only time your car was an issue or obstruction to the process then your conclusions as to the depth and scale of the problem may be very different to the previous case where the depth of problem is slightly greater. It may be that you conclude that this disastrous morning was just a chance event and not symptomatic of any greater issues. Essentially, joining together multiple cases allows us to be proportionate in our responses and ensure our action plans and improvements consider the whole system of safety rather than just one snapshot in time.

Returning to patient safety, triangulating and aggregating incidents relating to the same system of safety can provide an insight into the parts of the system that are failing and why. If incidents pertaining to the same system, all with individual insights with varying impacts on patient care, are aggregated, then we would be able to appreciate in what context a part of a system or process fails and how this affects other interconnecting parts of the system. This is almost akin to providing an insight into a stress test of a system — with the focus on how resilient the components of the system are in different contexts.

## When to Do a Thematic Review?

Whilst the previous section has identified the argument for thematic reviews, there is an important consideration as to when a thematic review is a useful and necessary investigatory approach. Thematic reviews of patient safety incidents can be used in any context of patient safety if they are reviewing the same system of safety. As described above, thematic reviews offer an opportunity to appreciate the complexity of a particular system of safety and, therefore, offer the most opportunity for learning when they cover the same portfolio or focus. For example, doing a thematic review of five cases, which include a fall, a pressure ulcer, a deteriorating patient, a dose omission and a delayed discharge, will not aid your understanding of the work system as they all focus on different safety systems, and it will not aid your understanding of the scale of the problem as they all relate to different safety systems. Some specific portfolios that benefit from thematic reviews include falls, pressure ulcers, deteriorating patients, medication errors, maternity specific incidents and diagnostic errors. These types of portfolios will allow you to appreciate the whole system of work and identify any areas where the controls lack resilience and/or are fallible to failure in certain circumstances and contexts.

The use of thematic reviews within patient safety investigation can be proactive or reactive. Thematic reviews can be a routine and proactive approach applied to a specific portfolio that we know is a high incident type in an organisation; for example, falls or pressure ulcers. In this proactive use of thematic reviews, it may be that this investigatory method is routinely conducted once a month, quarterly or annually for a local area, like a ward, or across several wards. Using thematic reviews in a reactive way sees us responding to a cluster of incidents that have occurred across the same portfolio over a particular period of time, for instance over the last two months. Using the organisation's incident management system may highlight to clinical leaders and patient safety a new emerging trend or theme and, therefore, a thematic review may be useful to appreciate the scale and complexity of the problem. An example of this type of use may be a recent trend of critical drug omissions (for example, Parkinsons, antiretroviral, or diabetes specific medication that cannot be omitted) across a group of inpatient wards.

## How to Do a Thematic Review of Patient Safety Incidents

### Who Should be Conducting Thematic Reviews?

The purpose of a thematic review is to gain an insight into a complex system of work and, therefore, it is important the review team have individuals who have expertise in the clinical system of work and in the principles of systems thinking. Those skilled in the particular system of work in focus will be able to make sense of the variability and complexities of systems and, crucially, provide insight into why processes may, rightly or wrongly, deviate from the work as imagined (e.g. policies, SOPs). Those skilled in systems thinking and the fundamentals of safety science will be able to guide investigations using a systems focus and a focus on resilience and system fallibility rather than be person-focused.

## What Data Can be Used Within a Thematic Review of Patient Safety Incidents?

It can be common for analysis to only use incidents recorded on the incident management system used by an organisation. This implicitly makes sense, but it is based upon the assumption that all safety records, events and insights are collected via incident reporting. There are commonly reported issues with barriers to incident reporting and the reporting culture of healthcare does not follow standards seen across other safety critical industries, for example aviation, which has been argued to have a better reporting and blame free culture (Kapur *et al.*, 2015). Therefore, we must be cautious about *only* using incidents as our window into safety issues and norms. If we consider thematic reviews as an opportunity to get closer to the realities of work, then we must make sure that the data we are using is representative of the work as done in the system of work. One of the most useful process steps to a thematic review can be utilising and triangulating different forms of data to help appreciate the whole work system.

Types of data that could be included in thematic reviews are:

- Incident records
- Complaints
- Narrative data (e.g. obtained from interviews or focus groups)
- Observational data (e.g. through ethnographic non-participant/participant observations)
- Inquest data
- Local reviews of care (e.g. perinatal mortality review tools (PMRT) or mortality and morbidity (M&M) meetings led by clinicians)
- Other data routinely collected (e.g. situational judgement reviews and audit)

## What are the Minimum Data Standards for Inclusion in a Thematic Review?

The data selected for inclusion in a thematic review must be reliable enough to base analysis upon. This is another reason triangulation of incidents is so important and validation of data from local teams. Once the data you have is of a quality that is good, the next key step is ensuring that you are able to compare the data in a systematic way. All the data types above are different forms of data and insight and, therefore, comparing and analysing them directly may be confusing and challenging because the information will not follow a standardised format. Getting the data ready for analysis is a key step to thematic analysis and a helpful tip may be imposing some sort of matrix on all data to analyse. This matrix could include key foci for the system of work and how it has been operationalised in each case. We could take the work as imagined or work-as-prescribed for the system of work and impose key questions onto the data to ensure that we can compare across our incidents. In the context of a cluster of medication safety incidents, our analytical matrix for the data we have could focus on these steps:

- The prescription stage (who prescribed it, where was the decision made, were there any difficulties or nuances in the prescription process, e.g. support needed?).
- The dispensing stage (who dispensed it, were there any variations to process?).
- The medication reconciliation stage (where drugs are reviewed and validated by a pharmacy professional) (what was the pharmacist's role in the process, was the medication reconciliation carried out?).

- The administration stage (how was the drug second checked, where in the process were there omissions?).
- Other (any information that is relevant to the system of safety, for example insights from patients or families).

Our data to analyse may focus on four incidents, a complaint, some observations, and a local audit. With this data, the investigatory team would need to sit down and relook at the data in the context of these five stages and questions. Much like thematic analysis as described in qualitative data methods, it is useful for these stages to be done independently by individual team members and then the findings brought together to be sense checked and shared. This part of the process tries to ensure that the data included in the analysis is following a set structure and that the analysis is based upon the system of work you are analysing.

An important note here is that the data you have may not have the detail or information you need and, therefore, some more data collection may be needed. This could be in the form of an AAR to ensure the thematic review has the correct and relevant depth of information to it.

## How Can Data be Analysed?

Data can be analysed both inductively and deductively. Once you have completed the step above and you are focusing on imposing a group of questions on your data before analysis, then this is referred to as deductive analysis as you already have a focus set and an analytical framework. If you were to just analyse the data as it was extracted and not place it into a specific format or answer specific questions, then this would be erring towards an inductive analytical technique. Deductive analysis is placing an already established framework to analyse within this framework. Inductive analysis involves not imposing any framework or structure to analysis and is commonly referred to as 'letting themes emerge from the data'. This will mean identifying links and cross cutting themes within the data as it is presented, rather than looking for specific foci based on an imposed matrix or framework.

## How Many Incidents or Cases Do I Need to Include in the Thematic Review?

This is a common question and, similarly to the evidence from thematic analysis research in qualitative research, there is no minimum number of cases to include. However, there is a practical consideration. Thematic reviews of patient safety incidents in this chapter are being argued to provide insight as to the depth of a problem and, therefore, including too many incidents may provide a great breadth of analysis rather than depth. As such, investigatory teams will need to ascertain what this balance is in the context of the safety system they are analysing. A thematic review with 11 cases to analyse will mean that the overall analysis will provide excellent insight into the spread or breadth of issue, but it may not identify the nuances of why certain processes, or parts of a work system, are failing in certain circumstances. Similarly, a thematic review of 3 cases may give excellent understanding of the depth of issue in terms of a detailed understanding of the dichotomy between the work as imagined versus the work as done but it may not help an investigatory team appreciate the full scale of a problem. However, anything between 3 and 12 cases is a pragmatic approach as long as the investigatory team is aware of the caveats above.

## How Long Does a Thematic Review Take?

There is no set length for how long a thematic review should take but there are key steps that will vary in length dependent on the scale of the problem, the complexity of the safety system in question and the number of cases you are analysing. The key steps to a thematic review include: (i) identification of a safety concern; (ii) sampling of data relevant to the safety concern; (iii) mapping the work system and creation of matrix (based on work as imagined/prescribed) and analysis, and; (iv) identification of learning and recommendations. These steps will vary in terms of time taken to complete and also be dependent on external factors e.g. time available to analyse data in conjunction with clinical roles and responsibilities.

## Example of How a Thematic Review Can be Used

Here is a fictious worked example of a thematic review of six cases of post-partum haemorrhage (PPH). Two of them are no harm cases, three are moderate harm cases as they resulted in interventional treatment to correct the blood loss, and one is a low harm event as it resulted in extra observation to the mother. There is also some data provided by a recent simulation-based training *in situ* around management of PPH. To start, we need to identify the work system for identification and management of PPH. The project team get to work, and they identify the below system of work:

- Risk assessment of women at risk of PPH completed and actioned appropriately.
- The routine method of collecting information on bleeding.
- The mode of ascertaining the blood loss volume.
- The escalation process dependent on the blood lost.
- Management of bleeding (e.g. within ward setting or escalation to theatre).

Now that the project team have this system of safety mapped out, they will need to ascertain if they have enough information in the incident cases to go straight into analysis of the data, based on these five stages. In this example, three out of the six cases had a local review done on them that can be used for the analysis; the other three have very scant detail included. Therefore, for the three incidents without much detail, all of which happened in the last six weeks, the team must go and complete AARs, or a form of local review, to ensure all six cases have the same level of information.

Once all six incidents have the same level of investigation and information, the analysis stage can start. Each of the six incidents can now be analysed across the five stages already identified. We may choose to do this inductively, and simply analyse all the data we have for each of the five stages. For example, in the context of the fourth stage in the system of safety, the escalation process, we may group together all information we have across the six incidents which pertain to the escalation process. We could choose to analyse each stage of the system deductively and create certain questions or subsections in each stage to impose on the data. For example, in the context of the fourth stage in the system of safety, we may have certain questions we want answered in terms of the escalation process:

- How much blood was lost before medical help was sought?
- Who contacted the medical help?
- What grade doctor was contacted?
- What decisions did the doctor make? How did they prioritise when to attend the patient?
- How quickly did it take the doctor to arrive at the patient's location?

The difference between inductive and deductive analysis in this example is that the latter type of analysis is imposing these questions on the data, rather than allowing the data to identify what the issues and learning points were (inductive). Once all stages of the safety system have been analysed in the context of the six incidents, the key learning points and findings can be displayed. Throughout this thematic review approach, the project team has been able to identify how the system of work has operated in the six individual cases and have identified any commonalities in system failures across this sample of data. An action plan with recommendations would then be completed as a result of this thematic review completed by the team. The recommendations from the review would be focused on the whole system and the complexity of the particular safety system. This is in comparison to a single investigation into the higher harmed case, which will note why the system failed for that particular individual case and, therefore, create recommendations based on that sole case. A thematic review in this example allows proportionate recommendations based on parts of the system that the review identifies to have fallibilities or lacking resilience rather than focusing on one case.

# Final Thoughts

This chapter has focused on the impact that thematic reviews can have for patient safety as we move towards embedding systems thinking into our everyday understanding of a safety and investigatory approach. The arguments for thematic reviews over single case investigations have been discussed, as well as providing a basis for the practical considerations of how to do a thematic review. While thematic analysis and reviews in the context of qualitative research is well established as a research method, its use within patient safety is an evolving portfolio. Research exists identifying its potential benefits and the methodology that can be followed (Machen, 2023), but research into its impact on safety and quality outcomes is limited. What is clear is that patient safety is moving towards systems thinking to ensure that learning is based on safety science principles and moving away from person-centered fallibility.

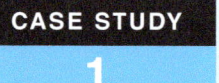

Andy Wilmer, Associate Director of Patient Safety, King's College Hospital NHS Foundation Trust

## Background

In early 2022, a decision was made at my organisation to trial the use of thematic reviews as a response to patient safety incidents.

We agreed to carry out trust-wide thematic reviews for key cross-cutting patient safety issues identified within our organisation. These were not necessarily areas of particular concern for the Trust (although some were), or emerging/escalating issues based on insight or triangulation but were based on backlogs of open incidents that previously we would have done RCA investigations into.

From a patient safety perspective, we hoped thematic reviews would help us to:

1. Support PSIRF implementation across the organisation through:
   a. trialling thematic reviews as a proportionate system-based approach to learning from patient safety incidents.
   b. introducing system-based proportionate approaches to responding to patient safety themes around the SEIPS framework as promoted by PSIRF (see also Chapter 3 on SEIPS).
   c. introducing the triangulation of different sources of insight into safety issues.
2. Identify systems-based insight into system safety vulnerabilities across the organisation.
3. Identify opportunities to improve patient safety.

From the organisation's governance/regulatory perspective, it was felt thematic reviews could also support:

1. Incident management across the organisation, particularly with the backlogs built up during the pandemic, through reducing the need for multiple similar investigations across different care groups into the same issues.
2. The completion of the outcome stage of the Duty of Candour regulations (again with backlogs of overdue cases built up because of the pandemic). Duty of Candour requires healthcare providers to operate in an open and transparent way with people receiving care or treatment.

When something unexpected or unintended occurs during their treatment, resulting in significant harm, it requires specific processes to be followed. Although this was well embedded in terms of initial transparency at the time a patient safety incident was identified, Duty of Candour requires us to keep patients updated on our inquiries into the event and this is particularly challenging when processes to carry out these inquiries (i.e. investigations) are resource heavy and capacity is limited (Care Quality Commission, 2022).

Thematic reviews were chosen as a methodology which could attempt to fulfil all the aims above — using a systems-based approach, proportionately, that could cover multiple (hundreds) of patient safety incidents.

## What We Did

This was a very new approach to safety for the organisation. Although previously aggregated reports of similar cases had (occasionally) been carried out, they were still based on RCA methodologies, individual chronologies and identification of care and service delivery problems.

Steps taken (although these generally emerged rather than being planned from the outset) were:

1. **Data analysis:** I manually analysed over a thousand open patient safety incidents to identify meaningful themes that could lend themselves to thematic review. This involved reading each of the incident reports and theming them based on my experience and expertise in patient safety. Although they were already categorised within our incident management system, the categories available generally added little insight because they were too broad (treatment, assessment, communication, etc.). Through this manual analysis, I identified around 20 cross-cutting high-level themes, each broken down into sub-themes, with data on which clinical areas they predominantly related to, to aid further analysis.

2. **Designing a methodology and template:** A group of patient safety leads and advisors were commissioned to research different approaches to carrying out thematic reviews while step 1 was carried out. At the time no nationally agreed template or guidance was available. The methodology developed included an attempt at systems-based analysis of the incidents (using SEIPS), a comparison of work as imagined (based on Trust policy/national guidance) and triangulation of insight from other sources (both internal and external). While an initial template was agreed, it did evolve iteratively as we undertook further thematic reviews. Subsequent to this work, guidance around the use of thematic reviews has been published nationally as part of the PSIRF learning response toolkit.

3. **Commissioning and prioritising the reviews:** Based on the analysis above, 16 thematic reviews were commissioned and conducted by the Patient Safety Team, Clinical Safety Team and Women's Health Quality, Safety and Governance Team. These were prioritised generally in order of how many patient safety incidents fell in each theme.

    Each review was carried out by a team of around four people to distribute the workload and to encourage team working and input from multiple perspectives. Subject matter experts and interested safety committees were identified for each review to provide additional insight and oversight.

4. **Systems-based analysis:** This was our first attempt at systems-based analysis and using the SEIPS framework so it took some adjustment. Previously, incident investigations had focused around 'what went wrong' with inconsistent analysis of why. Conclusions would often be 'failure to escalate, failure to order a pressure relieving mattress', etc., which led to weak and inappropriate improvement plans.

5. **Triangulation of insight sources:** Again, it was a fairly novel approach for the Patient Safety Team to be looking at anything other than incidents. We identified numerous sources of insight based on internal quality data (complaints, Patient Advice and Liaison Service (PALS), legal, risk, etc.) and external sources (HSIB, Getting It Right First Time (GIRFT), etc.). Data capture, analysis and triangulation was very challenging due to how internal information was recorded — often leading to searches based on keywords rather than a structured categorisation. However, we were able to draw key and recurring issues and system vulnerabilities from these sources.

6. **Drawing conclusions and recommendations for improvement:** Conclusions were drawn based on the above steps. We attempted to present these in a SEIPS format, breaking down the key safety challenges and system vulnerabilities relating to the theme under each system factor.

    We then made some guiding recommendations on how these could be explored further and where quality improvement or transformational work could be carried out.
7. **Governance and oversight of completed reviews:** Once completed, the thematic reviews were presented at a weekly panel meeting we started. Thematic reviews covering serious incidents were also taken to our Serious Incident Committee. These meetings allowed for discussion and scrutiny on both the approach taken and the findings.

    In some cases, improvement recommendations were incorporated into improvement plans/projects for Trust-wide safety workstreams. This worked particularly well for our Harm Free Care areas (e.g. falls and pressure ulcers). Other areas had less clear governance/workstream ownership to take forward findings.

    Following approval, processes around incident management could begin — that is, the organisational focus on closing incidents and the Duty of Candour processes.

## Lessons Learned

### What Went Well?

- We had positive senior buy-in from the outset, both from our Trust Executive and Integrated Care Board (ICB). Feedback on the reviews was overwhelmingly positive, with multiple requests for us to share our examples and experience with other organisations. Our ICB was more than happy to accept thematic reviews instead of individual serious incident reports in a proportionate, pragmatic and PSIRF style.
- Harm Free Care related thematic reviews were quickly incorporated into ongoing improvement work resulting in changes to our incident response for these types of issues that generally relate to the same small number of system vulnerabilities.
- The team approach to leading the thematic reviews was generally positive and created a more collaborative team dynamic compared to our historic care group-based structures.
- The team were agile in iterating their own processes as they learnt to carry out thematic reviews and use SEIPS on the job. Later reviews began to incorporate other methodologies, such as observational studies, rather than being primarily desktop-based reviews.

### What Didn't Go Well?

- There was no organisational plan for how improvements could be delivered based on systems analysis. There was concern around what the 'action plan' was and who was 'owning' delivery of any recommendations. However, this did lead to a wider review of safety improvement processes and governance structures.
- We had a 'work as imagined' barrier to how incidents would be managed and Duty of Candour fulfilled following the thematic reviews. There was a lack of understanding of how, when and why to use thematic reviews to support closure of incidents locally, and considerable barriers to their use to fulfil Duty of Candour (which had often been started more than a year earlier). There were unclear plans and unrealistic expectations that thematic reviews would be a panacea for incident management issues (i.e counting how many incidents were open/overdue).
- Where Duty of Candour was completed, there was negative feedback from patients/families about the impersonal nature of the response (and how it was delivered). This links to wider issues around how candour was carried out and the ongoing involvement of patients/families in responses. Patients often had unanswered specific questions to their case and were not particularly interested in how we were analysing themes at a wider level.

## Evaluation and Impact

The thematic reviews were successful against our initial patient safety aims. They were effective in providing insight and identifying opportunities for improvement in a systems-based and proportionate way. Resource has been shifted from low value-added activities, such as repetitive investigations, into known issues and weak actions. However, there has been no evidence on whether this has led to an increase in resources for compassionate engagement and improvement activities. The thematic reviews were effective for demonstrating SEIPS approaches to learning from patient safety events and how triangulation of insight sources can provide a greater understanding of contributory factors.

A systems-based approach, particularly at a thematic level, supports just and restorative practices as part of the organisation's safety culture. Through looking at safety themes at a wider level, and by looking at similar issues occurring in multiple different areas of the organisation, a focus on systems rather than individuals was demonstrated.

Processes to support improvement work in response to findings need to be strengthened — including organisational capabilities and resources to drive sustainable and effective improvement, and the governance and oversight functions.

Thematic reviews have been less successful at delivering some of the organisation's governance aims. Although the majority of patient safety incidents are now managed in a more timely and effective way — without the need for lengthy and limited value-adding investigations and development of often ineffective action plans — using thematic reviews to support this has been inconsistent across the organisation. There are variables around governance maturity, Care Group governance support and competing clinical demands.

There has been little to no impact in addressing concerns and risks around completion of the Duty of Candour outcome stage, with further resources and processes needed to support this.

## Conclusions

Agree clear aims and scope from the outset. Avoid trying to cover multiple aims, which can be contradictory. Ring-fence the aims that will give safety insight and inform and drive safety improvement. Perspectives on the success and effectiveness of thematic reviews in our trial differ based on perceived importance of the different multiple aims and created obstacles to the completion of reviews.

Thematic reviews are not helpful as the sole response to an incident. In our case this was unavoidable, but going forward I would use thematic reviews as an adjunct response periodically as a way of evaluating the impact of ongoing safety improvement work into known safety themes, and to understand whether any new sub-themes or contributory factors have emerged.

Where thematic reviews overlap with notifiable incidents under the Duty of Candour regulations, our experience is that thematic reviews are not appropriate as the sole response output a patient or family will receive. Going forward we will be recommending that all Duty of Candour incidents require a compassionate engagement response to ensure people affected (staff, patients and families) are supported in a transparent way and that questions are answered. This should fulfil the Duty of Candour steps where further learning response is not indicated (i.e. the contributory factors are understood and relate to already completed thematic reviews). People affected can be informed that a thematic review covering the incident may also be carried out to further inform improvement, with the opportunity for them to be involved in that if desired.

Carrying out a thematic review in a system-based way was challenging where there was no systems-based response to individual incidents to triangulate. This is something to consider when developing incident response plans. While an individual learning response may not be indicated for themes that have ongoing effective improvement work (e.g. falls), they may be helpful for carrying out periodic thematic reviews.

## Reflections from the Frontline

- The case study demonstrates the need for an organisational plan for how improvements could be delivered based on systems analysis. It is important to clarify who will 'own' delivery of any recommendations, and how the themed review will lead to wider review of safety improvement processes and governance structures. There needs to be clear plans and realistic expectations on how thematic reviews are going to help solve incident management issues.
- It is important to get buy-in from the outset from senior Trust staff and those from ICBs, Executives and Non-Executives, so they are prepared to receive thematic reviews. This is a significant change from the previous way of receiving individual serious incident reports.
- A key difference between theory and practice is that it can be challenging to look at patient safety insight in isolation. There are competing demands and priorities (e.g. governance/regulatory/risk-based aims), which may clash with the aims of curiosity and systems thinking. Providing the organisation with a detailed breakdown of system insight into one or many safety issues is not necessarily helpful without the appropriate improvement and assurance processes to do something about it.
- There needs to be better understanding of how, when and why to use thematic reviews to support closure of incidents locally, and considerable barriers to their use to fulfil Duty of Candour (which often may have been started more than a year earlier). This links to wider issues around how candour is carried out and the ongoing involvement of patients/families in responses. Patients often had unanswered specific questions to their case and may not be particularly interested in how an organisation is analysing themes at a wider level.
- There may be concerns that if patients and families don't receive sufficient personalised information from an incident specific review, they may be dissatisfied and seek more information through other sources, such as making a formal complaint. This may have significant implications for families and their confidence that the healthcare system is responding to their personal needs for information and justice. It may also lead to longer response times if a complaint is made as additional reviews will be needed. The resource implications of these will need to be factored in too.

## References

Braun, V. and Clarke, V. (2006). 'Using thematic analysis in psychology' in *Qualitative Research in Psychology*, 3(2): pp. 77–101.

Care Quality Commission (2022). *Regulation 20. Duty of candour.* https://www.cqc.org.uk/guidance-providers/regulations-enforcement/regulation-20-duty-candour.

Doupi, P. (2009). *National Reporting Systems for Patient Safety Incidents. A review of the situation in Europe 13.*

Health and Safety Executive (1999). *The cost to Britain of workplace accidents and work-related ill health in 1995/96.* Bootle: Health and Safety Executive.

Kapur N. *et al.* (2015). 'Aviation and healthcare: a comparative review with implications for patient safety' in *JRSM Open*, 7(1).

Machen, S. (2023). 'Thematic reviews of patient safety incidents as a tool for systems thinking: a quality improvement report' in *BMJ Open Quality*, 12:e002020. Doi: 10.1136/bmjoq-2022-002020.

Macrae, C. (2015). 'The problem with incident reporting' in *BMJ quality & safety*, 25(2): pp. 71–5.

Olsen, S. *et al.* (2007). 'Hospital staff should use more than one method to detect adverse events and potential adverse events: Incident reporting, pharmacist surveillance and local real-time record review may all have a place' in *Quality & safety in Health Care*, 16: pp. 40–4.

Shojania, K. (2009). 'The frustrating case of incident-reporting systems' in *Quality & safety in health care*, 17: pp. 400–2.

Stavropoulou, C., Doherty, C. and Tosey, P. (2015). 'How Effective Are Incident-Reporting Systems for Improving Patient Safety? A Systematic Literature Review' in *The Milbank quarterly*, 93(4): pp. 826–66.

Thomas, E. and Petersen, L. (2003). 'Measuring Errors and Adverse Events in Health Care' in *Journal of general internal medicine*, 18: pp. 61–7.

CHAPTER 11

# Conclusion

*Claire Cox, Jordan Nicholls and Helen Hughes*

Our aim in producing *Patient Safety: Emerging Applications of Safety Science* has been to bring together different practical examples of the latest approaches being used to carry out expert and compassionate patient safety investigations, designed to help improve care and treatment and prevent avoidable harm.

The true test of impact in learning from incidents and applying that learning will be service improvement and the future reduction of avoidable harm. The incredible contributors to this book — the academics, researchers, patient safety managers and others that gave freely their time and insights — are committed to supporting this improvement journey. We will continue to collaborate and drive change.

*Patient Safety: Emerging Applications of Safety Science* has taken as its basis for this the NHS's new PSIRF. As discussed in the introduction, PSIRF promotes a range of system-based approaches for learning from patient safety incidents (NHS England, 2022). The contributors to this book have focused on providing insights and suggestions on the use of practical safety tools for review and improvement associated with this new framework.

By its nature, this book provides only snapshots of tools and experiences in practice and is not intended to provide a comprehensive summary of how to undertake forensic incident investigation. Nor does it replace the need for experienced, qualified and compassionate investigators. However, it does offer a range of different reflections from academics and practitioners alike of the application of safety science, systems theory and NHS policy into practice.

As far as we are aware, this is the first 'how to' guide developed for practitioners and organisational patient safety leaders on the potential for improving how the NHS approaches developing and maintaining effective systems and processes for responding to patient safety incidents. As mentioned in the Foreword of this book, Ted Baker notes that improvements to patient safety are often incremental and built on 'a consistent implementation of the best safety practice, with healthcare at last coming to terms with the risks inherent in its ever-increasing complexity'. In this spirit, we hope that this book will prove to be a useful resource for those on this journey to improve patient safety and reduce avoidable harm, both in the UK and globally.

We hope that the approaches, insights, tools and advice provided in this book will help address these implementation challenges and that learning will lead to action and improvement. We recommend this book to everyone who has a role in transforming patient safety throughout the healthcare system.

We have learned in developing this book that there is much interest and commitment to applying the principles for PSIRF as part of this journey; a journey that unites clinicians, patient safety experts, patients and families, academics, researchers, policy makers, media commentators, politicians and the general public. The challenge, as with many patient safety initiatives, is one of implementation (Patient Safety Learning, 2022). Healthcare struggles to consistently translate patient safety insights and learning into practical improvements, often as a result of:

- An absence of a systemic and joined-up approach to safety.
- Poor systems for sharing learning and acting on that learning.
- Lack of system oversight, monitoring and evaluation.
- Unclear patient safety leadership.
- A poor culture with organisational priorities that don't place safety as a core purpose.

The importance of sharing and acting on learning from using new incident investigations techniques and tools is something that is a high priority for members of the Patient Safety Management Network (PSMN). As mentioned in the Introduction, much of the impetus for this book has evolved from discussions from the PSMN, an informal voluntary network, created by and for patient safety managers, and hosted on Patient Safety Learning's online platform, *the hub* (Cox, 2023). Members of this Network have highlighted the importance of having the resources available to guide their organisations in implementing PSIRF.

It is important that going forward, the implementation and effectiveness of PSIRF is properly evaluated. Indeed, some evaluation work has already commenced (University of Leeds, 2022). Going forward it will be invaluable to understand:

- How well the PSIRF initiative has been disseminated and understood by organisational and patient safety leaders, as part of an explicit programme of work to improve organisational culture.
- The development of organisational PSIRF policy and plans across all organisations that provide NHS-funded care.
- Whether the new tools and approaches are supporting more systems-based insights and learnings in incident investigation.
- Whether patients and their families are being engaged and supported.

Sir Liam Donaldson (2022) said in his report *Organisation with a Memory*, 'To err is human, to cover up is unforgivable and to fail to learn is inexcusable.'

It is inexcusable that our health systems are not adequately learning and avoidable harm continues across our organisations and health systems. The intention of PSIRF is to support learning and application of that learning. We hope that this book contributes to the effective implementation of PSIRF.

The true test of PSIRF and other patient safety programmes will, of course, be the implementation of service improvements that reduce avoidable harm.

Supporting the PSMN and the authors in coming together to compile this book is Patient Safety Learning, a UK-based charity and independent voice for improving patient safety. On *the hub* (www.pslhub.org), their award-winning platform to share learning for patient safety, there is an ongoing process to support and share improvements in incident investigation, including:

- Hosting the PSMN and providing a safe space for weekly drop-ins for people working in patient safety in the UK, with PSIRF implementation being a topic of regular discussion (Cox, 2023).
- Collating PSIRF plans and resources on *the hub* (Patient Safety Learning, 2023a, 2023b & 2023c).
- Sharing knowledge and good practice on *the hub*.
- Awareness raising and campaigning of the importance of organisational leadership engagement with safety as a core purpose.

The incredible contributors to this book, the members of the PSMN and Patient Safety Learning will continue to collaborate and drive change and ensure that we learn and apply learning for improvement. Please join us on this improvement journey by joining *the hub*, and if your work in the UK involves patient safety, please do join the PSMN weekly drop-in sessions and community forum.

# References

Cox, C. (2023). *The voices of the patient safety frontline — the Patient Safety Management Network two years on*. Patient Safety Learning, *the hub*. www.pslhub.org/learn/professionalising-patient-safety/the-voices-of-the-patient-safety-frontline--the-patient-safety-management-network-two-years-on-r9894/.

Donaldson, L. (2022). *An organisation with a memory*. Clinical Medicine Journal, 2(5): pp. 452–7.

NHS England. *Patient Safety Incident Response Framework*. www.england.nhs.uk/wp-content/uploads/2022/08/B1465-1.-PSIRF-v1-FINAL.pdf.

Patient Safety Learning (2022). *Mind the implementation gap: The persistence of avoidable harm in healthcare*. https://www.patientsafetylearning.org/blog/mind-the-implementation-gap-the-persistence-of-avoidable-harm-in-the-nhs.

Patient Safety Learning (2023(a)). *Patient Safety Incident Response Plan (PSIRP) finder*. https://www.pslhub.org/learn/investigations-risk-management-and-legal-issues/investigations-and-complaints/methodology-and-guidance-how-to-do-an-investigation/patient-safety-incident-response-framework-psirf/patient-safety-incident-response-plan-psirp-finder-r10372/.

Patient Safety Learning (2023(b)). *Top picks: PSIRF insights and opinions*. https://www.pslhub.org/learn/investigations-risk-management-and-legal-issues/investigations-and-complaints/methodology-and-guidance-how-to-do-an-investigation/patient-safety-incident-response-framework-psirf/top-picks-psirf-insights-and-opinions-r10249/.

Patient Safety Learning (2023(c)). *Top picks: PSIRF tools, templates and examples*. https://www.pslhub.org/learn/investigations-risk-management-and-legal-issues/investigations-and-complaints/methodology-and-guidance-how-to-do-an-investigation/patient-safety-incident-response-framework-psirf/top-picks-psirf-tools-templates-and-examples-r10248/.

University of Leeds (2022). *The Response Study*. https://responsestudy.leeds.ac.uk/.

# Index

## A

AcciMaps, 113–124
    case studies, 125–135
    construction of, 114
Active self-learning, 80
ActorMaps, 124
After Action Review (AAR), 14, 79–88
    case studies, 88–92
    components of, 82–87
    conductor, 84–85
    ground rules, 85
    implementation, 87
    legal issues, 87
    origins of, 79–80
    patients and family members as participants in, 86
    purpose of, 83–84
    quality issues, 87
    research, 86–87
    theory, 80–81
Agency for Healthcare Research and Quality (AHRQ), 12
*An organisation with a memory*, 1
Appreciative Inquiry (AI), 7
As low as reasonably practicable (ALARP) principle, 66

## C

Change management
    application of, 12–14
    components, 14
    examples of, 11–14
    framework, 14
    outside of healthcare, 6–7
    within healthcare system, 7–8
Chartered Institute of Ergonomics and Human Factors (CIEHF), 69
Clinical Negligence Scheme for Trusts (CNST), 72
Code of Practice (2020), 53
Community care, 50
Compensation Act 2006, 50
Compounded harm, 3, 44
Comprehensive Unit-based Safety Program (CUSP), 12–13
Crew Resource Management (CRM), 24

## F

Fishbone diagram, 25
Functional Resonance Analysis Method (FRAM), 68

## G

General Medical Council (GMC), 87
Global Patient Safety Action Plan, 3

## H

Halligan, Aidan, 80
*Handbook for Evidence Implementation* (Porritt), 8
Healthcare
    change management in, 7–8
    engagement lead, 47–50
    history of, 5
    impact of, 50
    moral duty, 43
    proactive safety in, 3–4
    restorative approach, 57–58
Healthcare Safety Investigation Branch (HSIB), 46, 54
Health Foundation, 9

Heinrich, Herbert, 156
Heinrich's Domino model, 65
Hierarchical Task Analysis (HTA), 99
Hollnagel, Erik, 66–67
Human Factors Analysis and Classification System (HFACS), 125
Human Factors and Ergonomics (HFE), 19, 95
  transformative simulation and, 141–142

I

Insight strategy, 2
Instantaneous Self-Assessment Method (ISA), 141
Institute of Medicine, 1

J

Joint cognitive systems, 66

K

Kotter's eight-step change model, 7

L

Leadership, 11
Learning healthcare system (LHCS), 8
Learn together programme, 50–52
Leveson's STAMP model, 67
Lewin's planned change theory, 6
Lippitt's phases of change theory, 6
Litigation, impact of, 50

M

Maternity care, 50
Memorandum of Understanding (MoU), 54
Mental health, 50
Multi-agency healthcare, 50

N

National Police Chiefs' Council (NPCC), 54
National Policing Improvement Agency (NPIA), 54
National Safety Standards for Invasive Procedures (NatSSIPs) Network, 3
National Training Centre (NTC), 80
*NHS Patient Safety Strategy* 2019, 2, 43
Nursing and Midwifery Council (NMC), 87

O

Organisation for Economic Co-operation and Development (OECD), 9

P

Paediatrics, 50
Parliamentary and Health Service Ombudsman (PHSO), 44
Patient and Family Liaison Officer (PFLO), 48, 49
Patient safety
  case study, 58–61
  defined, 1
  engaging patients for, 3
  examples of change management and, 11–14
  healthcare simulation, 139
  importance of, 44
  improving, 9–11
  involvement, 45–53
  needs of, 43
  in NHS, 1–2
  patient and family engagement, 41
  practical tools, 2–3
  resilience, 67
  restorative approach, 57–58
  Safety-II, 65–72
  simulation in, 141
  system-level challenges, 52–53
  thematic reviews in, 155–162
Patient Safety Incident Response Framework (PSIRF), 2
Patient Safety Learning (2022), 3
Patient Safety Management Network (PSMN), 2, 170
Patient Safety Partners Network, 3
Performance Influencing Factors (PIFs), 97–99
Performance variability, concept of, 67
Plan, Do, Study, Act (PDSA) cycle, 8
Prison healthcare, 50

Q

Quality improvement (QI), 11–12

R

Rasmussen, Jens, 66
Reason's Organisational Accident model, 65
Risk, 66
Rogers' diffusion of innovation theory, 7

S

Safety-I, 2, 65
Safety-II, 2, 65–72

applying, 68–70
case study, 73–76
challenges in, 70
definition of, 67
example of application of, 70–72
need for, 66
performance variability, 67
Strengths, Weaknesses, Opportunities and Threats (SWOT) analysis, 143
Swiss Cheese model, 65
System Engineering Initiative for Patient Safety (SEIPS), 3, 8, 19–40, 83
application, 26–27
and basic systems thinking principles, 24–25
case studies, 28–38, 98–99
examples, 20
framework, 20–22
introduction, 19
multi-functionality examples, 23–24
patient perception, 125
system assumptions of, 25
*vs.* fishbone diagram, 25
worksheet, 22
work system, 21
Systems-Theoretic Accident Model and Processes (STAMP), 67

## T

Team Based Quality Review, 79
Thematic analysis, 155
argument for, 156–158
case study, 162–165
example of, 161–162
of patient safety incidents, 158–161
use of, 158
Transformative simulation, 139–141
application, 143–146
case study, 146–151
HFE and, 141–142
taxonomy, 142–143

## W

Walk-Through-Talk-Through (WT3) analysis, 95, 96
advantages&disadvantages, 102
application, 99–100
benefits of, 96–97
case study, 103–107
example, 101
usage, 100–101
Woods, David, 66
World Bank, 9
World Health Organization (WHO), 3, 9
World Patient Safety Day, 3